# THE
# PATH *to* LOVE

# Books by DEEPAK CHOPRA

—◆—

Creating Health

Return of the Rishi

Quantum Healing

Perfect Health

Unconditional Life

Ageless Body, Timeless Mind

Journey into Healing

Creating Affluence

Perfect Weight

Restful Sleep

The Seven Spiritual Laws of Success

The Return of Merlin

Boundless Energy

Perfect Digestion

The Way of the Wizard

# THE
# PATH *to* LOVE

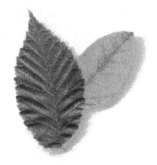

Renewing the Power of Spirit
in Your Life

# DEEPAK CHOPRA

*Harmony Books*
NEW YORK

Grateful acknowledgment is made to the following for permission to reprint copyrighted material: For *Birdsong* by Rumi, translated by Coleman Barks. Copyright © 1993, Coleman Books, Maypop. • From *Rabindranath Tagore: The Myriad-Minded Man* by Krishna Dutta and Andrew Robinson. Copyright © 1995 by Krishna Dutta and Andrew Robinson. Reprinted by permission of St. Martin's Press Paperbacks. • From *Crazy as We Are* by Rumi, translated by Dr. Nevit O. Ergin. Published by Hohm Press 1992. • From *W. H. Auden: Collected Poems* by W. H. Auden. Copyright © 1940 and renewed 1968 by W. H. Auden. Reprinted by permission of Random House, Inc., and Faber and Faber Ltd. • From *Feeling the Shoulder of the Lion* by Rumi, translated by Coleman Barks. Copyright © 1991. Reprinted by permission of Threshold Books, R.D. 4, Box 600, Putney, VT 05346. • Excerpts from "The Upanishads," "The Odes of Solomon," and "Symeon the New Theologian" from *The Enlightened Heart* by Stephen Mitchell. Copyright © 1989 by Stephen Mitchell. Reprinted by permission of HarperCollins Publishers, Inc. • Excerpt from page 122 ("The Cloud of Unknowing") from *The Enlightened Heart* by Stephen Mitchell. Copyright © 1991 by Stephen Mitchell. Reprinted by permission of HarperCollins Publishers, Inc. • The Acorn Press, Durham, N.C., for permission to quote from *I Am That: Talks with Sri Nisargadatta Maharaj,* translated by Maurice Frydman, edited by Sudhakar S. Dikshit (9th printing, 1996).

Published by Harmony Books, a division of Crown Publishers, Inc., 201 East 50th Street, New York, New York 10022. Member of the Crown Publishing Group.

Random House, Inc. New York, Toronto, London, Sydney, Auckland

http://www.randomhouse.com/

Harmony and colophon are trademarks of Crown Publishers, Inc.

Design by Lynne Amft

Printed in the United States of America

Library of Congress Cataloging-in-Publication Data is available upon request.

ISBN: 0-517-70622-9

10  9  8  7  6  5  4  3  2  1

First Edition

# CONTENTS

# ACKNOWLEDGMENTS

Writing a book about love is a unique challenge, in both heart and mind, and from the outset I realized that it would have to be born in an atmosphere of love. Some other people understood this as well, and it is to them in particular that I owe deepest gratitude.

To Peter Guzzardi, whose sensitivity and nurturing went far beyond the duties of an editor—you opened the way and kept it open against all odds.

To Patty Eddy and Tina Constable, who stand behind the scenes at Harmony Books and accomplish wonders.

To my agent Muriel Nellis, godmother to my whole career as a writer.

To my support staff at The Chopra Center for Well Being and Infinite Possibilities International, especially to David Simon, Richard Perl, Deepak and Geeta Singh, Roger Gabriel, and Arielle Ford —without your loyalty and immense enthusiasm, I would not have found the opportunity to write this book at all.

And, as ever, to my family, who walk the path to love with me, no matter what turn it takes.

*EVERYTHING IN THE UNIVERSE
IS WITHIN YOU.
ASK ALL FROM YOURSELF.*

*—Rumi*

# THE
# PATH *to* LOVE

# 1

# REVIVING
# A LOVE STORY

$A$ll of us need to believe that we are loved and lovable. We began
life with confidence on both points, bathed in a mother's love and
swaddled in our own innocence. Love was never in question, but
over time our certainty clouded. When you look at yourself today,
can you still make the two statements every infant could if it had the
words?

> I am completely loved.
> I am completely lovable.

Few people can, for looking at yourself honestly you see flaws that
make you less than completely lovable and less than perfectly loved.
In many ways this seems right to you, for perfect love is supposedly
not of this world. Yet in a deeper sense, what you call flaws are really
just the scars of hurts and wounds accumulated over a lifetime. When
you look in the mirror, you think you are looking at yourself realisti-
cally, but your mirror doesn't reveal the truth that endures despite all
hurt:

# THE PATH *to* LOVE

*You were created to be completely loved and completely lovable for your whole life.*

In a way it is amazing that you do not realize this, because underneath everything you think and feel, innocence is still intact. Time cannot blemish your essence, your portion of spirit. But if you lose sight of this essence, you will mistake yourself for your experiences, and there is no doubt that experience can do much to obliterate love. In an often hostile and brutal world, maintaining innocence seems impossible. Therefore, you find yourself experiencing only so much love and only so much lovability.

This can change.

Although you perceive yourself in limited terms, as a mind and a body confined in time and space, there is a wealth of spiritual teaching that says otherwise. In spirit you are unbounded by time and space, untouched by experience. In spirit you are pure love.

The reason you do not feel completely loved and completely lovable is that you do not identify with your spiritual nature. Your sense of love has lost one thing it cannot afford to do without: its higher dimension. What would it be like to restore this lost part of yourself?

> *Mind, body, and spirit would unite—this union creates the love you have to give.*
>
> *You and your beloved would unite—this creates the love you have to share.*

In our deepest nature each person is meant to be the hero or heroine of an eternal love story. The story begins in innocence, with a baby's birth into a mother's loving arms. It proceeds through stages of growth, as the young child steps out into the world. With more and more experience the circle of love widens, including first family and friends, then intimate partners, but also taking in love of abstract things, like learning and truth. The ripening journey brings us to love of giving, and the blossoming of higher values, such as compassion, forgiveness, and altruism. Finally there is the direct experience of spirit itself, which is pure love. The journey climaxes in the same knowledge that a baby began with, although it couldn't voice that knowledge: I am love.

*You know that you have fully experienced love when you turn into love—that is the spiritual goal of life.*

Not many people find the spiritual goal of life. The aching need created by lack of love can only be filled by learning anew to love and be loved. All of us must discover for ourselves that love is a force as real as gravity, and that being upheld in love every day, every hour, every minute is not a fantasy—it is intended as our natural state.

This book is about reviving love stories that should never have faded. The union of self and spirit is not only possible but inevitable. The spiritual meaning of love is best measured by what it can do, which is many things.

Love can heal.
Love can renew.
Love can make us safe.
Love can inspire us with its power.
Love can bring us closer to God.

Everything love is meant to do is possible. Knowing this, however, has only made the gap between love and non-love more painful.

Countless people have experienced love—as pleasure, sex, security, having someone else fulfill their daily needs—without seeing that a special path has opened to them. Socially, the "normal" cycle of love is simply to find a suitable partner, marry, and raise a family. But this social pattern isn't a path, because the experience of marriage and raising a family isn't automatically spiritual. Sad to say, many people enter lifelong relationships in which love fades over time or provides lasting companionship without growing in its inner dimension. A spiritual path has only one reason to exist: it shows the way for the soul to grow. As it grows, more of spiritual truth is revealed, more of the soul's promise is redeemed.

When you find your path, you will also find your love story. People today are consumed by doubts about their relationships: Have I found the right partner? Am I being true to myself? Have I given the best part of myself away? As a result, there is a restless kind of consumer shopping for partners, as if the "right" one can be found by toting up a potential mate's pluses and minuses until the number of pluses matches some mythical standard. The path to love, however, is never about externals. However good or bad you feel about your relationship, the person you are with at this moment is the "right" person, because he or she is a mirror of who you are inside. Our culture hasn't taught us this (as it has failed to teach us so much about spiritual realities). When you struggle with your partner, you are struggling with yourself. Every fault you see in them touches a denied weakness in yourself. Every conflict you wage is an excuse not to face a conflict within. The path to love therefore clears up a monumental mistake that millions of people make—the mistake that someone "out there" is going to give (or take) something that is not already yours. When you truly find love, you find yourself.

Therefore the path to love isn't a choice, for all of us must find out who we are. This is our spiritual destiny. The path can be postponed; you can lose faith in it or even despair that love exists at all. None of that is permanent; only the path is. Doubt reflects the ego, which is bound in time and space; love reflects God, eternal divine essence. The ultimate promise on the path to love is that you will walk in the light of a truth extending beyond any truth your mind presently knows.

I have structured the following chapters to lead the reader anew on the path to love, from the first stirrings of romance to the final stages of ecstasy. Falling in love feels like an accidental occurrence to many people, but in spiritual terms it is not—it is the entrance point to love's eternal journey. Romance has several distinct phases for us to explore—attraction, infatuation, courtship, and intimacy—each partaking of a special spiritual significance.

In the dawning of the next stage, romance turns into a committed relationship, usually marriage, and the path changes. Falling in love is over; being in love begins. Spiritually, the word *being* implies a state of the soul; it is this state that a couple learns to nurture through surrender, the key word in every spiritual relationship. Through surrender the needs of the ego, which can be extremely selfish and unloving, are transformed into the true need of the spirit, which is always the same—the need to grow. As you grow, you exchange shallow, false feelings for deep, true emotions, and thus compassion, trust, devotion, and service become realities. Such a marriage is sacred; it can never falter because it is based on divine essence. Such a marriage is also innocent, because your only motive is to love and serve the other person.

Surrender is the door one must pass through to find passion. Without surrender, passion is centered on a person's craving for pleasure and stimulation. With surrender, passion is directed toward life itself—in spiritual terms, passion is the same as letting yourself be swept away on the river of life, which is eternal and never-ending in its flow.

The final fruit of surrender is ecstasy: when you can let go of all selfish attachments, when you trust that love really is at the core of your nature, you feel complete peace. In this peace there is a seed of sweetness perceived in the very center of the heart, and from this seed, with patience and devotion, you nurture the supreme state of joy, known as ecstasy.

This, then, is the path to love outlined in the following pages, although it isn't the only one. Some people do not fall in love and enter into relationships with a beloved. But this does not mean that there is no path for them, only that the path has been internalized. For such people, the Beloved is entirely within themselves from the very outset. It is their soul or their image of God; it is a vision or a calling; it is a solitariness that blossoms into love for the One. In its own way, such a love story is also about relationship, because the final realizations are the same for all of us. To realize "I am love" is not reserved only for those who marry. It is a universal realization, cherished in every spiritual tradition. Or to put it most simply, all relationships are ultimately a relationship with God.

I wanted this to be a practical work as well as, hopefully, an inspiring one. Each chapter includes exercises (titled "Loving Practice") that will enable you to ground yourself in the insights discussed in the text. Following this comes a love story (titled "In Our Lives") to amplify the text in a more personal way. I am involved in all these stories, usually as a sympathetic listener to friends, patients, and fellow seekers. Sometimes I step beyond that role to function as counselor or adviser, but I do not set myself up as a professional therapist. I only want to open the way to insight, acting as its mid-wife; it is up to every person to actually give birth.

But before embarking on the love stories in this book, let me tell a bit of my own. Spirit is always leaving clues about its existence, although we may not be on the lookout for them, and I remember the first clues given to me by my cosmic grandmother. She was my paternal grandmother, married to an old sergeant in the Indian army who had blasted his bugle from the rooftops the morning I was born. To look at her, this tiny woman didn't appear cosmic. Her idea of contentment was to pat flour dough into perfectly round bread for my breakfast or to wend her way before dawn to a dim temple where the thousand names of Vishnu were chanted. But one day, as I sat waiting by the charcoal stove for my breakfast *paratha* stuffed with potatoes and spice, she let me in on a piece of cosmic wisdom.

We had a neighbor down the street in the cantonment of Poona, a Mr. Dalal, whom nobody liked. He was stooped and gray, very thin, and he greeted everyone with a sour, pained expression. Curiously, he had a small, vivacious wife—his exact opposite—who adored him. They were always together, and if I happened to pass them on the way to school, Mrs. Dalal would wave to me from underneath her blue sari, all the time keeping a loving eye on her husband, who would be tapping his way down the sidewalk with his cane.

"They are like Rama and Sita," my grandmother said admiringly behind their backs. This I very much doubted, since Rama and Sita were divine incarnations of man and woman, and the most perfect lovers in Indian mythology. When Rama strung his bow it caused lightning and thunder, while Sita was beauty itself. Being eleven and obsessed with cricket, I had little time for either Rama and Sita or the Dalals, until a shadow passed over our household. Mr. Dalal lay dying just a few doors away from us.

My grandmother paid a visit to his bungalow and came back looking somber and pale. "Only a few hours," she told my mother. Small boys can be callous about death, and I resented Mr. Dalal for the time he had poked his cane at me and ordered me to pick up a package he had dropped on the sidewalk. Years later, when I had entered medical school, I realized that Mr. Dalal had been suffering from angina, and his weak heart had not permitted him even to bend over. Severe chest pain accounted for the twisted expression on his face, and now it had brought him to death's door.

Of course Mr. Dalal's dying was the talk of the neighborhood. That day my grandmother informed us that Mrs. Dalal had decided to die in her husband's place. She was praying fervently for this wish. Our family was stunned, except for my father, who was a cardiologist. He kept quiet, only assuring us that Mr. Dalal had no hope of recovery from his infarction. A week later this prediction was confounded when an extremely frail Mr. Dalal and his wife appeared again on the street. Mrs. Dalal, very much alive, waved from beneath her blue sari, looking as cheerful as ever, if somehow changed.

My grandmother waited, and only a few months passed before Mrs. Dalal fell sick. A minor cold turned to pneumonia, and in those days when penicillin was not so readily available or believed in by common people, she died, suddenly, in the middle of the night.

"Like Rama and Sita," my grandmother murmured, wearing a look on her face that could be mistaken for triumph. She described the last scene between husband and wife, when Mr. Dalal took off his prayer beads and laid them tenderly around his wife's neck before she passed. "That is a real love story," she said. "Only love can work such a miracle."

"No," I protested, standing impatiently by the stove. "Mrs. Dalal is dead. You call that love, but now they both have nothing." My father had already told me, in his measured, clinical voice, that Mr.

Dalal's survival had been a fluke, not a miracle. He could be expected to die within the year.

"You just don't understand," my grandmother reproached me. "Who do you think gave Mrs. Dalal her wish? When she loved her husband, she was loving God, and now she is with him. Every real love story is a love story with God."

An old woman with a cosmic mind is a good place to begin to talk about love. For this story isn't about Mrs. Dalal. A Westerner would be skeptical that she had achieved anything of value by dying for her husband, assuming that was what had happened. The point of the story lies in my grandmother's deepest beliefs:

> *A man and a woman can reflect divine love in their love for each other.*
>
> *Loving your beloved is the way you love God.*
>
> *Human love survives death.*

If you could hold the same beliefs, your love would contain a profound power and meaning. Actually, I shouldn't deprive Mrs. Dalal of her own meaning. The neighbors whispered that she was murmuring "Rama" when she died. Anyone who can say God's name at such a moment might well be wooing her lover. Looking back, I now realize that for her, death itself was a healing. How many modern people in the West can say the same?

Despite the fact that love is important to everyone, few of us could deny that love is in a crisis—no deeper crisis exists. Either love isn't a powerful enough force to save us from our darker nature or something has happened to turn us away from love. Perhaps love was never the answer we were looking for.

Any of these possibilities could be true. If they are, however, to be human is truly tragic. In his last major work, *Civilization and Its Discontents,* Sigmund Freud painted a picture of human nature that is grimly unloving. Humans, he asserted, are motivated by an instinct for sexual gratification that society can barely keep in check. They are born to take sadistic satisfaction in the plight of enemies; they will use ruthless violence to obtain money, power, and sex; and only the threat of retribution from someone more powerful keeps this violence in check. According to Freud, Christ's injunction to love thy neighbor as thyself is a psychological impossibility.

Every adult has seen enough of life to agree at least partially with this devastating assessment, and modern psychology, by and large, is based on it. The famous Milgram pain experiments from Yale in the 1950s demonstrated that when ordered to give electric shocks to strangers in a laboratory setting, average people would follow such orders willingly, even when the subjects screamed in agony and begged them to quit. Where is love in all of this?

> *The direct experience of spirit is the only lasting foundation for love.*

Despite all the evidence to the contrary, in some profound way we were created for love to the very depths of the human soul. This spiritual vision of human nature has prevailed against all odds. Its roots go back in India more than two thousand years to the Vedic scriptures. *Veda* is Sanskrit for "truth" or "knowledge." The hymns of the Rig Veda are considered to be humanity's oldest devotional expression, but as it expanded into thousands and thousands of scriptures, Veda continued to emphasize the same point: the human being is a mirror of God. Our being and God's Being are one.

In the Vedic view we are not passive observers of reality but creators, as God is. The mask of matter disguises our true nature, which is pure awareness, pure creativity, pure spirit. Like light streaming from a bonfire, reality streams from us, and our choice is to emanate love or non-love. Contrary to Freud's dark view, the Vedas say that it is much more natural for us to create from love than non-love. They declare that humans "are born in bliss, sustained in bliss, and return to bliss again after death." This is a drastic shift in perception from modern psychology, and yet to be truly in love always brings a new perception—everyone can validate the sudden ecstasy and bliss that makes romance so sweet. But to have a complete vision of love means being willing to undergo a much more total shift of perception.

> *When you perceive yourself as spirit, you will not simply feel love—you will be love.*

In spiritual terms, to be love is only natural. It is our departure from love that is unnatural. The ancient scriptures recognized man's violence and saw it clearly: one of the most important teachings of Veda is the *Bhagavad-Gita,* which is set on a battlefield before a murderous war. Yet in the Vedic tradition an unbroken succession of saints, seers, masters, and sages have seen beyond violence and ex-pressed themselves as follows:

> Life is love and love is life. What keeps the body together but love? What is desire but love of the self? . . . And what is knowledge but love of truth?

The means and forms may be wrong, but the motive
behind is always love—love of the me and the mine.
The me and the mine may be small, or may explode
and embrace the Universe, but love remains.

The voice is that of a South Indian master, Nisargadatta Maharaj, speaking to followers in the late 1970s. The expression "life is love and love is life" has such ancient roots that no idea is more venerable. Yet this is a love we have lost contact with in our own age, distracted as we are by sexual attraction, unstable emotions, and religious dogma. Love based on the experience of spirit gives rise to the possibility that we can return to our true nature, throwing aside our unloving behavior as a bad and very long dream.

A love based on "higher" values espoused by the world's religions seems, as Freud pointed out, impossibly ideal. The scriptural injunctions to love the Lord with all thy heart, all thy soul, and all thy might are legion. Yet there is sober truth in Emily Dickinson's mournful little poem:

Sometimes with the Heart
Seldom with the Soul
Scarce once with the Might
Few—love at all.

If all our attempts to find a spiritual foundation for love have shown themselves to be so wanting, where can we turn?

Spirit can only be called on when it is real, and it can only be real if it is real *for you*. In other words it has to *be you*. This is exactly what the Vedas teach. Rather than "soul," they equate spirit with "Self," not the everyday self with its thoughts, wishes, needs, and drives but a higher Self that is silent and eternal. The difference is explained in a classic Vedic metaphor: every person is like a piece of gold. If you were a gold ring, a gold watch, a gold chain, you could say "I am a ring, a watch, a chain," but these are temporary shapes. In truth you are just gold—that is your essence, no matter how the shape changes.

In the same way, we each have a self, defined in modern psychology as an image developed over time. It is a mysterious fusion of ego, personality, and memory that everyone amasses between infancy and early childhood. Being completely personal, your self is also completely isolated and separate from every other self. Yet, if you saw yourself truly, you would no longer identify with this haphazard, ramshackle thing, your self. In truth you are the Self, created from the same spirit that in infinite form is called God. You are one grain of gold, compared to which God is all the gold that exists, and yet you can rightfully say, "I am gold."

> *We all draw upon the higher Self for identity, life, awareness, will, and love.*

The Self that Lord Krishna teaches about in the *Bhagavad-Gita* is an eternal aspect of human nature that transcends all individuality, all change in time and space. Speaking of the immortal "dweller in the body," Krishna declares,

> Weapons cannot cut him,
> Fire cannot burn him,
> Water cannot wet him,
> Wind cannot blow him away. . . .
> He is eternal and pervading everything,
> Subtle, immovable, and ever the same.

What is important here is that the Self is a *real experience*. It is not an ideal, far removed from ordinary reality—which is how most of us think of the soul—but as close to you as breath. The Self is love's source, and therefore it is more real than the things that block love—anger, fear, egotism, insecurity, and mistrust. Those qualities, however widespread they may be in society, are temporary; they grow up over time and have to be learned. The Self, by contrast, is secure in peace and safety; it knows only love because its experience is only of love.

When you interact with another person, you are free to feel anything, from the deepest hatred to the deepest love. You may be repelled or attracted; you can convey rejection or acceptance. But at the level of the Self, you always meet another person in love.

> *The person you love reflects your share of universal love. If you learn to look deep enough, you will see that your reality is only love.*

In a famous passage the Vedas declare,

> As is the microcosm, so is the macrocosm,
> As is the atom, so is the universe.
> As is the human body, so is the cosmic body,
> As is the human mind, so is the cosmic mind.

This verse can be simplified to a few words: you are the universe. Whatever a person sees in his or her surroundings, from the smallest detail to the largest panorama, *is* that person. Reality is a mirror of the soul.

The Vedic tradition divided the world into reality and illusion. Illusion, or *Maya,* is composed of transient forces and events. Reality is formed of spirit. Thus the task set for every person was to pierce the veil of illusion in order to discover the spirit in everything. The same task is set before us now.

Materialism has no room for an assertion like that. After having written more than a dozen books about the conjunction of mind and body, which seemed radical a few years ago, I now find myself witness to the weakness of materialism on all fronts. What is a healing prayer but a successful attempt to abolish the distinction between inner and outer reality? What is a spontaneous remission of cancer but the material body's obedience to wisps of intention entertained by the mind? Einstein's physics tells us that everything that appears solid to our senses is actually 99.999 percent empty space. The classic Eastern metaphysical description of a spiritual reality standing behind an empty material illusion suddenly seems very plausible.

My cosmic grandmother was the person who taught me that the angels eternally pull against the demons. In her worldview the angels always win—the world of love is ultimately the one we are born to live in. My experience has also given me hope that this is true, and out of that hope I decided to write this book about love.

Darkness, however terrible, never fully extinguishes the spark of light. One of the most moving love stories I've ever read happened between two enemies in the Holocaust. A devout Catholic was suffering in a hideous medical "experiment" being conducted at Auschwitz. She was a young woman, and as it happened the doctor who presided over her clinical torture was also a woman, which somehow made her sadism all the more horrifying. Death came slowly, but at last it came. The young woman whispered unintelligibly, and the doctor, assuming she was uttering a curse, drew back.

The young woman reached out. She struggled to lift something from her neck and managed at the last moment to hold it out to her tormentor. "For you," she was whispering as she handed her rosary to the doctor, a last blessing as she departed the world.

Such a story arouses a surge of hope amidst the tears. We would all like to believe that one redeemed soul can help redeem another, even in the depths of terrible darkness. If that is true, then love's power is as great as spiritual teaching tells us it is.

I am not proposing in this book that we simply go back in time and adopt Indian metaphysics—that would be impossible, given the vast changes in culture over the past few thousand years. Instead I propose that the Vedic sages were the first to map a path to love, which they called a *Sadhana*. A path implies a beginning and an end. In this case the beginning is a reality in which love is longed for but uncertain, swamped by fear and anger, overwhelmed by the counterforce of hatred. The end is a reality where nothing exists but love.

*What remains now is the deepest healing of all, the healing of love.*

# LOVING PRACTICE

## Making a Soul Bargain

Healing the split between love and spirit is the goal of this book, and periodically I will give practical suggestions to that end. Usually these "loving practices" are directed to the reader, but I recommend, where possible, that you and your beloved both try them.

The first loving practice addresses doubts you may have about whether a "higher" love has any kind of accessible reality. To someone who has never fallen in love, you cannot prove that the experience exists. There is no power in words to evoke passionate romantic love, just as the fragrance of a rose is meaningless however beautifully you describe it. How much more alien, then, is the love promised by union with spirit? Look at the following list of things that love is supposed to accomplish, expanded from the list that appeared earlier in the text:

> Love is meant to heal.
> Love is meant to renew.
> Love is meant to make us safe.
> Love is meant to inspire us with its power.
> Love is meant to make us certain, without doubt.
> Love is meant to oust all fear.
> Love is meant to unveil immortality.

Love is meant to bring peace.
Love is meant to harmonize differences.
Love is meant to bring us closer to God.

Even if this list strikes you as unrealistic, or wildly overblown, I want you to make a bargain with love—a soul bargain—*that any or all of these things will come true for you.*

Take a piece of paper and write down what you want from love. If it is a real force, if it is attuned to who you are, love will respond. Make your list as complete and specific as you can. I suggest writing down every entry from the preceding list and beside it just what you want. For example:

*Love is meant to heal.*

I want to heal my anger toward my father. I want to heal the love I couldn't give to my children when they needed it. I want to heal my hurt over losing my friend *X*.

*Love is meant to renew.*

I want to feel renewed enthusiasm for my work. I want to renew the sexual feelings I have for my wife. I want to renew my sense of being young.

*Love is meant to make us safe.*

I want to feel safer with other people. I want to feel safe when I go outdoors for my morning run. I want to feel safe from having *X* reject me if I tell him I love him.

*Love is meant to inspire us with its power.*

I want my love to be powerful. I want to use all my own power with love. I want to express love when I feel it and not give in to lower emotions like fear and anger.

Once you are satisfied that you have detailed everything you want —and don't feel afraid to ask too much—the bargain is complete. Put the piece of paper away in a safe place. You have announced to your soul what you want, and it is up to love to respond. Love is intelligent and aware; it knows you better than you know yourself. Therefore it has the power to fulfill its side of the bargain. Rest easy and be attentive over the next few months. Don't dwell on your list or try to make it come true. There is nothing you need to do except this:

> *When you feel love, act on it. Speak your heart. Be truthful.*
> *Remain open.*

This is how you align yourself with love. At the end of a few months, take out your list and read it over. Ask yourself how much has come true. I won't say that you will be amazed at what love has actually done—although many people are—but you will certainly be surprised. Actually asking for love is one of the most difficult things for anyone to risk, and by risking it first in your heart, you open a door that will never close again.

# IN OUR LIVES

## There's Somebody Out There

"I know what you're thinking," Delaney said. "You think I'm too choosy, right? But I don't think I'm asking that much. It's not that she has to be drop-dead gorgeous or a Ph.D."

"You just have standards," I suggested.

"Right. I think of it as a package. If the whole package is right, the details don't matter all that much."

"Assuming that she, whoever she is, likes *your* package," I said. Delaney nodded. He was amazingly immune to irony, and I knew it wasn't fair for me to aim it at him. He really did want to fall in love —it was his biggest goal in life—and since Delaney had succeeded at all his other goals, it was frustrating how elusive this one was turning out to be. Once he and I had done a residency together in Boston, where he had been raised in a working-class family, and we later moonlighted at the same suburban emergency room to make ends meet. It had been fifteen years since he set up his cardiology practice, and only now, in his midforties, did Delaney feel he could make time to find a mate. It was hard for him to hide how confused about it he was in his own mind.

"Thank God I'm not one of those guys who's dumping his wife of thirty years for a sexy twenty-something girlfriend," he said. "For me this is a fresh start. I'm optimistic, I'm patient, but I guess—"

"What?" I asked.

Delaney looked away, a faint cloud of doubt on his face. "I don't know. Maybe I'm too old," he muttered.

"Or too demanding," I said. "Isn't a sexy twenty-something part of the package you're looking for? Be honest."

He shrugged sheepishly. "A guy can hope."

I felt a sudden uneasiness about Delaney and his newest project, immediately followed by a wave of sadness. The fact that our culture teaches us so little about love was staring me in the face. We had been talking about a man's "love life" for an hour, and yet we hadn't touched on anything even remotely resembling love.

"Have you ever fallen in love before?" I asked. "Really fallen?" Delaney looked startled, apparently not expecting our conversation to get this personal. He hesitated.

"Well, I'm not coming from nowhere on this thing," he said. "I've had some really sweet times, and lots of women want to go out with me." I nodded.

"Listen, we don't have to go anywhere you don't want to go," I said quietly. "But I think you're feeling a little lost." He stiffened, and I could see him retreat inwardly. I said, "That wasn't an accusation. It's natural to feel lost. Especially if you're not looking in the right places."

"I hate the places where I go," he said angrily.

"The bars? Everyone hates those places," I said. "But that's not what I meant. You're not looking in yourself—that's the place where she is, whoever you hope to find." Delaney stared at me as if I was indulging in paradox, but I pressed on. "You've had a lot of accomplishment in your life, and basically you've used the same approach every time. You see a challenge, you muster your resources, and with enough confidence and self-assurance you win what you're after. That's right, isn't it?" He agreed. "Accomplishing anything important involves risk," I said, "and therefore fear. But if you let the fear dominate, you'd never take any risks, and therefore you wouldn't accomplish anything."

"Are you saying I'm afraid to fall in love?" he asked. "Then why would I be looking for it?"

"No, I'm not saying that," I replied. "But love and fear very often touch, and people like you, who have undertaken very difficult things—going to medical school on a shoestring, opening your own practice, raising money for expansion and new ventures—have to learn how to keep fear out of the picture. And not just fear— self-doubt, confusion, despair, hopelessness—most of the common human frailties, in fact. Keeping your frailties out of sight becomes extremely important if you want to amount to anything in this world, but that is exactly the opposite of what love demands."

Delaney flinched. I could tell he didn't like the word *demand*. "I have weaknesses, like everybody else," he said grudgingly. "What do you want me to do—go around parading how vulnerable I am so that some woman will take pity on me?"

"You're exaggerating because you hate the idea so much," I said. "No, you aren't out to attract pity. What I'm trying to get at is that 'normal' life requires everyone to appear as strong as possible, and this tactic, which may work in other areas, fails miserably when it comes to love."

Like most people, Delaney had never considered how his inner world was constructed, but everyone creates psychological divisions as a means of survival. We wall off inner compartments, and into them we shove all the undesirable things about ourselves—our secret fears, weaknesses, and flaws, our deep sense of doubt, our belief that we may be ugly or unlovable. Everyone has these dark chambers of the soul.

"Do you think you're lovable?" I asked Delaney.

"My God, what a question!" he blurted. "It's not anything I think about. I just want to get married, you know, like everyone else."

"That question would take most people aback," I said, "but why? Is it embarrassing to feel lovable? The discomfort arises because love can feel too personal, even for ourselves; it pokes into those compartments where our negative self-image is stored. Unfortunately, to fall in love means going there—that's what love demands."

True love is more dangerous than most people are willing to admit. It arouses the same discomfort as in dreams where you find yourself naked in a public place. If falling in love meant going into all the dark chambers of the soul, none of us would risk it. On the other hand, to love another person involves opening up your whole being. What makes the risk possible is the ingredient of spirit.

Spirit is the real you, beyond all divisions into good and bad, desirable and undesirable, lovable and unlovable. Love exposes this reality, which is why falling in love is a blessed state. For many people it is the only one they will ever know in a lifetime. The spiritual overtones of romantic love are unmistakable. First there is a tremendous emotional opening, a liberation. Your whole being flows toward your beloved as if the two of you share the same feelings, the same likes and dislikes, almost the same breath. The secondary effect of this inrush of delight is a release of cares and anxiety; the cloud of infatuation swallows up worries over such trivialities as money, career, and the fate of mankind. Even if you had no spiritual background at all, you would have tasted the soul's sweetness by falling in love. As the great Persian poet Rumi says,

> When love first tasted the lips
>  of being human,
> It started singing.

This blessing of falling in love comes from spirit, but it can be blocked by ego. Ego is responsible for protecting your self-image; it creates the compartments where everything undesirable about you has been hidden. What blocks love is not the presence of these shadow energies but the division of the psyche that came about when your ego started building inner walls. Love is a flow, and walls keep the flow out.

In spiritual terms, this is the problem of duality. By dividing good from bad, right from wrong, we essentially insist that parts of ourselves are unlovable—why else would we keep them out of sight? We turn ourselves into packages, exactly the kind Delaney talks about. The package seems to contain only good and worthy things, but if another person ventures to love us, the whole package spills open, and a lot of what it contains isn't so nice.

The cruelest consequence of duality is that we believe in the rightness of shutting love out. "Being open" is equated with "being weak." "Being closed" is equated with "being strong." And society reinforces these dualities by reminding us, day in and day out, that this is not a world where love is safe.

As with most people, I don't encounter much love except inside my home. On waking I see my wife's face beside me, and many mornings I marvel at the ineffable love this sight inspires, something far more delicate and moving than I can put into words. Yet beside my bed also lies the newspaper I read to get to sleep, and in it is all the hatred anyone could imagine. On every page I confront the catastrophic failure of love. There is personal failure in the overwhelming amount of divorce, litigation, and social bitterness we've learned to live with. There is public failure in the war, street crime, and oppression we all go to bed praying will not strike us.

Although no one can say where love went, it is a dangerous sign that we are surrounded by so many images pretending to be love.

Every day we are saturated, drowned with images of romance from books and films, bombarded with sex from advertisements, and goaded on all sides to become more attractive in order to win attention from a "perfect" lover. Delaney was struggling in the swamp of non-love, as we all are, trying to find something he really couldn't name.

"What if you sat down and imagined the perfect woman waiting out there for you," I told him. "You've probably done it many times, only to give up. Well, I think you're going to find that woman, and it will happen the instant you can let go of her image. It sounds like a paradox, but letting go has to be the first step in finding someone to love you, because love is never an image. Love doesn't depend upon external values at all."

"I know that," he said, with sudden and surprising gentleness. "I felt I had no choice but to have some kind of image in mind. Otherwise, it was like looking in the dark."

"Most people have that worry," I said. "It reflects their own secret belief that they are not all that desirable themselves, and also their fear of loneliness. At least they have an image to keep them company. There's a deeper issue here, though. Does love ever come from outside ourselves?"

"Of course it does," he said.

"Go into it more deeply," I urged. "All of us believe in duality, which creates the perception that people are separate. You and I seem separate, sitting here in this room. We have separate bodies, separate minds, separate memories and backgrounds. Separation is the foundation of our whole existence. But part of you hates living in separation—it hates the fear, loneliness, suspicion, and alienation that come with being totally isolated. This part of you calls upon love to solve its pain. If only you can find someone to love you, perhaps the separation will be healed."

"You don't make my life sound very pretty," Delaney mourned.

"No," I said. "But in their heart of hearts most people feel the pangs of separation; it's not a secret. Let me ask you, Do you really believe there's a perfect somebody out there waiting for you? As common as that myth is, the reality is different. The somebody waiting for you is always a reflection of yourself. Out of our loneliness, all of us seek a source of love that will fill up the lack we feel inside, and that's exactly what happens, no more and no less."

"I don't know how to respond to that," Delaney said.

"If you observe yourself closely enough," I said, "you'll see the patterns. Most men, for example, feel a lack of tenderness, which they hope to find in a woman. Most women feel a lack of strength, which they hope to find in a man. Whatever the need is, the person who fills it becomes the source of love.

"The question is, how do we keep this going? Can the person who happens to match our needs continue to make us feel loved? I don't think so. We all have too much hidden inside; there is too much healing to do. So in time the outside source of love fades; it stops being effective. And then certain truths dawn:

*"You can never receive more love than you are prepared to receive.*

*"You cannot give more love than you have to give.*

*"The love reflected from another person has its source in your own heart.*
The reason love from outside sources stops working is that you haven't solved separation, only papered it over."

"So then what?" he asked.

"You stand at a crossroads. You can go out again and search for love from some new source, you can make do with what you have, you can turn to satisfactions other than love, or you can be totally honest and give up the search for externals altogether."

Here we had reached a critical point. The path to love begins when you realize that separation, loneliness, and the pain of isolation are real. Not many people want to face this fact, and therefore they resign themselves to a sadly constricted amount of love. As a healer, love knows no limits, but you must be willing to bring your whole being to it. Only then does the balm of love flow.

"There's something I really admire in you," I told Delaney. "I think you'll be surprised what it is. You haven't settled for imitations. In some part of yourself, you are waiting for the real thing." Delaney met my eyes; he nodded ever so slightly. "It's such a hard thing to talk about," I said, "this nameless longing that only love can fill. What are we waiting for? What is the real thing, if not the flood of images about romance, sex, and endless pleasure that the ideal lover is supposed to gift us with? In reality we are the gift and we are the giver.

"Duality is and always has been an illusion. There is no one out there waiting for you. There is only you and the love you bring to yourself. In spirit you are united with all other souls, and the only purpose of separation is for you to rejoin that unity."

"Which makes love the only blessing," Delaney said quietly. We sat for a moment, letting his words sink in, for it was as if he spoke from my heart too. "Yes," I said. "Love is the only blessing, and that means all love. If love is the ultimate reality, as the great teachers tell us, then the slightest gesture of connection is a gesture of love. To reach across the wall of separation, whether to friend, lover, family, or stranger, is to act in the name of love, whether we consciously realize it or not."

We had reached a special moment, which we both wanted to appreciate in silence. We had been talking in Delaney's office in suburban Boston, an ordinary room, but for a moment not ordinary. The path to love always opens unexpectedly. Our world contains such chaos and confusion that it is a miracle there is a path at all. Yet as long as there is separation, there will be a bridge. "I think you've gotten at one of my secrets," Delaney said after a pause. "I had lost faith that anybody out there really would love me as much as I wanted her to."

"Love doesn't take faith," I said. "Because separation is an illusion, believing in *it* is what takes faith. Love is real. It can be held, nurtured, felt, learned from, and depended upon. So abandon your faith. Stop wishing and hoping, and turn your efforts to what is real. Duality is so flimsy that it is ready to fall apart at any moment. In our imaginations we believe that love is apart from us. Actually there is nothing but love, once we are ready to accept it."

# 2

# THE PATH

— 🌿 —

In the West what we generally call love is mostly a feeling, not a power. This feeling can be delicious, even ecstatic, but there are many things love is meant to do that feelings cannot.

*When love and spirit are brought together, their power can accomplish anything. Then love, power, and spirit are one.*

There has never been a spiritual master—not Buddha, Krishna, Christ, or Mohammed—who wasn't a messenger of love, and the power of the message has always been awesome: it has changed the world. Perhaps the very immensity of such teachers has made the rest of us reticent. We do not accept the power love can create inside us, and therefore we turn our backs on our divine status.

India is a society where every person is divine, but only a few realize it. Strangely, the same can be said of the West. The only difference is that you can see holy men bathing in the sacred rivers of India, while our holy men go unnoticed, hidden from sight in monasteries or the grave. "Let them be rich in the West," my friend Lakshman would say loudly. "There, saints have to be dead to be real. Ours are walking around outdoors!"

Outdoors, but not always that easy to find. Countless seekers have traveled through India without meeting any genuine saints. Or rather they did not perceive them to be holy. Thanks to Lakshman, a man who combines boisterous exuberance with deep reverence, I've had occasion to feel the presence of yogis and sages in their Himalayan caves or rickety wooden ashrams on the Ganges. Lakshman told me a story about how he gained his first belief in saints. We were sitting in a café in La Jolla, California, worlds away from our origins, watching the blue Pacific roll in the sun.

"For a long time, Deepak, I wasn't a believer in these so-called saints. Half of them are scoundrels, idle beggars wandering from door to door, taking advantage of people's innocent faith to get a handout. One suspects that the rest are probably psychotic. Or so I thought. My family in Bangalore is very Westernized; we started a computer software company ten years before the explosion of technology in South India. We keep up our daily *puja* prayers at the altar in the dining room, but it's a formality.

"I live in an old part of the city. From my window I can see medieval Shiva temples being blackened by fumes from thousands of scooter rickshaws and battered lorries. Old India and new India come together in a war zone of screeching sensory assault—that is what I wake up to every day.

"One morning I couldn't bear to fight the traffic, so I decided to walk to work. My parents' factory is not far from the center of town. You know how the sidewalks are in India—impossible! Ten minutes from home I was totally frustrated, pushing my way through a sea of peddlers, beggars, layabouts, and twenty thousand other working people trying to get to the same place I was. The image of a dry Ganges flowing with humanity came to mind. Well, it came to mind later, since all I felt at the time was irritation and exhaustion.

"Rounding a corner I saw a knot of people gathered around

something. Of course they blocked the whole sidewalk, and this being India, traffic had stopped while taxi and lorry drivers got out to have a look too. Something in me snapped, and I furiously pushed through, shouting for everyone to get out of my way. No one did. In five seconds I was embedded in a pack of shoving bodies, unable to escape.

"You can't imagine how it felt. Of course you can, having been there yourself. But there I was, on the verge of screaming, when I suddenly felt everything in my mind stop. My anger and frenzy, my preoccupations, the constant flow of associations—the whole baggage simply disappeared, leaving behind an empty mind. I'm no fool; I had read scriptures and knew all that stuff about an empty mind being the silence of God. But on the streets of Bangalore! Somehow I managed to push my way forward. There in the middle of the pack was a small woman in a white sari, sitting with her eyes closed. She must have been about thirty, I suppose, and something about her told me she was from a country village.

"To this day I have no idea why she had stopped in the middle of the sidewalk like that. She sat completely still, not minding the crush around her. Actually, the crowd was acting quite respectful on the whole; she was surrounded by a ring of people on their knees. I got a little nearer, and the most remarkable thing happened. My empty mind began to have something in it, not a thought but a sensation. *Mother.* That's the only way I can describe it. It was as if all the mothering feelings that women give to their families were inside me, but with much greater purity and clarity.

"I wasn't thinking of my own mother. There was just this feeling. It grew stronger, and I saw, like a revealed truth, that this woman on the sidewalk was emanating the energy of 'mother' from its very source. I also saw with complete clarity that my own mother had been trying to express this same energy. However imperfectly, she

31

was connected to a reality that doesn't depend on this mother or that mother. It is just 'mother,' the endless love of the feminine toward everything in creation.

"The next second I was on my knees, only a few feet from this saint on the sidewalk. She had her eyes open now and was smiling at all of us. Her smile somehow made my experience far more intense. I had a flashing glimpse of thousands upon thousands of souls wanting to be here on earth to experience the preciousness of being a mother.

"What came to me then was forgiveness: I realized that all the people who can't love, even the most evil and criminal ones, are trying to express this divine energy. We are all on the path, and despite our differences, being on the path makes us much more similar than we realize."

Lakshman's voice trailed off. Although his encounter had lasted only a few minutes, its effect was permanent. He remains awed that the mere presence of a saint can uplift ordinary awareness (this effect is called *Darshan* in Sanskrit). More important, he became convinced that a path to the divine is real, since he had now met someone who was at the end of that path.

I can speak from experience too. I never had the startling breakthrough Lakshman did, but my parents were devout, and my retired grandfather frequently spent his afternoons on the veranda soaking up the darshan of swamis and saints. A boy doesn't grasp much of the deeper meaning of such experiences; that came only when I was an adult, after sitting myself with strange, otherworldly recluses and feeling utterly loved in their presence.

Their surroundings were sometimes appalling, with nothing to eat or drink but a dipper of greenish water. There would often be no recognition that I had walked into the saint's presence, no smile or encouraging gesture. Yet the moment I closed my eyes, I was in a remarkable space. I had been welcomed to a dance, the play of the universe, which was taking place not as whirling stars and galaxies but in pure silence. A blissful coolness penetrated my body, and I lost awareness of the sticky shirt clinging to my back and the suffocating trapped air. The sensation was one of peace, but there was an extraordinary vibrancy to it, as if thrills of invisible energy were running through me. At times it was almost more than I could bear. My inner space seemed to be exploding. I was suspended in emptiness that was not empty but teeming with everything ever created or to be created —the womb of the cosmic mother. *And it was all in me.*

These are memories that make me sure that our current concept of love is not adequate. We all use the word *love* to mean many things, and to be in love is often a complex, confusing state. Yet what I experienced was incredibly simple:

*Love is spirit. Spirit is the Self.*

Self and spirit are the same. Asking "What is spirit?" is just a way of asking "Who am I?" There isn't spirit outside you; you are It. Why aren't you aware of It? You are, but only in a limited way, like someone who has seen a glass of water but not the ocean. Your eyes see because in spirit you are the witness to everything. You have thoughts because in spirit you know all. You feel love toward another person because in spirit you are infinite love.

Restoring the spiritual dimension to love means abandoning the notion of a limited self with its limited ability to love and regaining the Self with its unbounded ability to love. The "I" that is truly you is made of pure awareness, pure creativity, pure spirit. Its version of love is free from all memories or images from the past. Beyond all illusion is the source of love, a field of pure potential.

That potential is you.

# THE PATH *to* LOVE

## WHAT IS THE PATH?

The most valuable thing you can bring into any relationship is your spiritual potential. This is what you have to offer when you begin to live your love story at the deepest level. Like the seed needed to start the life of a tree, your spiritual potential is the seed for your growth in love. Nothing is more precious. Seeing yourself with the eyes of love makes it natural to see others that way too. You will be able to say of your beloved, as the poet Rumi does:

> You are the secret of God's secret.
> You are the mirror of divine beauty.

The path to love is something you consciously choose to follow, and everyone who has ever fallen in love is shown the first step on that path. The unfolding of spiritual potential has been the chief concern of all the great seers, saints, prophets, masters, and sages in human history. Theirs was a carefully charted quest for the Self, a far cry from our notion of love as a messy, emotional affair.

In India, as I've mentioned, the spiritual path is called *Sadhana,* and although a tiny minority of people give up normal life to wander the world as seekers of enlightenment (these are monks, or *sadhus*), everyone, from those in the most ancient civilization of Vedic India until today, considers their life to be a sadhana, a path to the Self. Although the Self seems separated from us, it is actually intertwined in everything a person thinks, feels, or does. The fact that you do not intimately know your Self is amazing, if you come to think about it. Looking for your Self, the Vedic sages declared, is like a thirsty fish looking for water. But as long as the Self has yet to be found, sadhana exists.

34

# The Path

*The goal of the path is to transform your awareness from separation to unity. In unity we perceive only love, express only love, are only love.*

While the inner transformation is taking place, every path must have some outer form to sustain it. In India a person's nature leads him to the style of path appropriate to reaching fulfillment. Some people are naturally intellectual and are therefore suited to the path of knowledge, or *Gyana*. Some are more devotional and are suited to the path of worship, or *Bhakti*. Some are more outwardly motivated and are suited to the path of action, or *Karma*.

The three are not mutually exclusive; ideally, one would include in one's lifestyle daily periods of study, worship, and service. All three approaches would then be integrated into a single path. It is, however, entirely possible to be so taken with a single approach that your whole existence may be centered on reading the scriptures, contemplation, and scholarly debate—the life of gyana. Or you may spend your time meditating, chanting, and participating in temple rituals—the life of bhakti. Or you could do social work, apply yourself to mental and physical purification, and do God's bidding in daily activity—the life of karma. Even in the most traditional sectors of India today, these paths have broken down, giving way to modern lifestyles in which study and work have little or nothing to do with spiritual aspirations.

What does this mean for a Westerner who has never been exposed to sadhana? I propose that being on the spiritual path is such a natural and powerful urge that everyone's life, regardless of culture, obeys it. A path is just a way to open yourself to spirit, to God, to love. These are aims we all may cherish, but our culture has given us no established, organized way to reach them. Indeed, never in history has a seeker been confronted with such a disorganized and chaotic spiritual scene.

What we are left with is relationships. The desire to love and be loved is too powerful ever to be extinguished, and fortunately a spiritual path exists based upon this unquenchable longing. The expression *path to love* is not simply a metaphor; it reappears throughout spiritual history in many guises. The most ancient version is the bhakti or devotional tradition from Vedic India, in which all forms of love ultimately serve the search for God. The Sufis of Islam have their own devotional lineage. Rumi, whom I quote so often, was more than a poet; he was a great teacher of this path. To him God was the sweetest, most desirable lover, whose touch he could feel against the skin:

> When it's cold and raining,
> You are more beautiful.
>
> And the snow brings me
> even closer to Your Lips.
>
> The Inner Secret, that which was never born,
> You are that freshness, and I am with You now.

Christ initiated another version of the path in his supreme teaching, "Love thy neighbor as thyself." Jesus always spoke of God as a loving father. The Christian version of the path is therefore a relationship not so much between lovers as between parent and child or a shepherd and his flock (we shouldn't forget, though, the image of Christ as bridegroom and the worshiper's soul as the bride).

So it isn't the tradition that is lacking. One might more fairly say that in most religions the teaching of love, as originally presented, seems to have faded, to have become more an ideal than a practical reality. But amidst all the confusion and breakdown of traditional teaching, there is still the spark of love that brings two people together, and out of that a path can be made.

Like the tiny spark of fire that consumes a forest, the spark of love is all you need to experience love in its full power and glory, in all its aspects, earthly and divine. Love *is* spirit, and all experiences of love, however insignificant they seem, are actually invitations to the cosmic dance. Within every love story hides the wooing of the gods and goddesses.

In a different age the most fleeting of infatuations had spiritual meaning; the nearness of God in the beloved was taken seriously. Since the advent of Freud, however, psychologists have assured us that falling in love is illusory; the sense of ecstasy that is part of falling in love isn't realistic. We must learn to accept the temporary nature of romance and disregard the "projected fantasy" that we might be as immortal and invulnerable as passionate lovers feel. We would therefore have to be skeptical of Walt Whitman when he rapturously declares,

> I am the mate and companion of people, all just as
>     immortal and fathomless as myself,
> (They do not know how immortal, but I know.)

And W. H. Auden would have to be seen as indulging in hyperbolic fantasy when he says, in the first rapture of love,

> . . . in my arms I hold
> The flower of the ages,
> And the first love of the world.

The sense of delight, uniqueness, and blessing felt by lovers has its own reality, but you must find it within. Romance and spirit are both states of inner truth. In this book I am proposing that the two can be joined. The dramatic psychological shift that occurs whenever we fall in love is actually *a temporary state of spiritual liberation, a glimpse of who you really are.* The ecstatic feelings that flow between lovers, their sense of being uniquely cared for and protected, their belief in a timeless state of being—all these are spiritual realities. The East has tended to retain the spiritual dimension of falling in love, even at its most passionate, as in this line from Rumi:

> Love is the way messengers
> from the mystery tell us things.

In this vision of love, which expands far beyond two people and their infatuation, the acts of love join us to a reality that we yearn for but do not know how to reach—the "mystery."

In this book I will use the phrase "spiritual master" to designate someone who has achieved command over spiritual reality. Despite the huge cultural differences between a Sufi master, a yogi, a Christian saint, and a Chinese martial artist of the highest proficiency, all can perceive spirit as clearly as you or I see the earth and sky. The spiritual masters were not idly setting forth idealistic goals when they taught the path to love. In a very practical sense the path enables two people to escape the trap of separation and suffering. In its place are peace and ecstasy. The freshness of life is love and nothing else. When two people can grow into that knowledge, the promise of lasting happiness becomes real.

# LOVE, PLEASURE, AND HAPPINESS

Naturally the question arises, "Why should I choose a path at all?" Relationship, with or without romantic love, has existed for a long time. Being in love with someone hasn't required making any conscious spiritual choices other than which church to go to, perhaps, and in the case of parenthood, what faith to raise the children in. Insisting upon the spiritual dimension of love may sound uncomfortably exalted to some people, who are content to enter a relationship for happiness and security. Therefore it's worth asking how happiness is actually achieved, and whether we can really attain security without embarking upon the spiritual journey.

On the surface the absence of spirituality seems to make little difference to what people perceive as happiness. I was surprised to discover recently that happiness is not a rare commodity. In opinion polls when people are asked if they are happy, roughly 70 percent say yes. This response is amazingly consistent. The same percentage holds for every age-group, from the very young to the very old. It does not vary widely from country to country or year to year. The one striking exception occurs among impoverished people. The very poor tend to be less happy, and in Asia, where vast numbers of people do not have their basic needs met, the pollsters' question "Are you happy?" is often met with a blank stare.

On the surface, then, love hardly seems indispensable given how many of us already say that we are happy. I think this is an example of a word that appears to be self-defining when it really isn't. "Happiness" is just as fluid as love itself and equally elusive. Outward conditions have no predictable effect on either. For example, people who have struggled out of poverty say that they are happier, but once people are above the poverty line, adding more money doesn't increase happiness. It often takes considerably more expense to provide a new stimulus, and without stimulus most people can't be happy.

In the long term, however, depending upon stimulus is a trap. Enough stimulus of the right kind may create happiness, but the balance is extremely precarious. Studies have shown that newborn babies, for example, like to have pretty dangling things in their surroundings. A mobile with ten shiny objects on it will cause a baby to gurgle and laugh when it's placed over the crib. However, if you take away eight of the dangles and leave behind only two, the baby will cry in loud protest.

This is probably the earliest experimental evidence we have that happiness is vulnerable to loss. Certainly we all grow up coming to this conclusion—deprive us of our money, our jobs, our relationships, and our quotient of happiness drops dramatically. Likewise we don't like to have our stimulus be out of control. Babies have been sat in front of screens that flash pretty pictures, which they can make come and go by pulling a string. Having this kind of control is very pleasing. But if the pictures come and go at random, the same happiness doesn't result. Worse still, if the baby pulls the string and nothing happens on the screen, he will be very unhappy. Again, this is a lesson we all learn—random events in our lives, or people who do not prove predictable, undermine our sense of control, leading to unhappiness.

What all this amounts to is that the word *happiness* too often means "pleasure response." All response depends upon stimulus, just as sexual pleasure depends upon being aroused and stimulated. This undeniable fact leads countless people to panic when their source of pleasure vanishes. Those of us who bounce from one failed marriage to another exhibit in full-blown form this craving for stimulus. But any desire to keep things smooth, predictable, and comforting has the same shadow hanging over it. There can be no sense of security in your existence when it depends upon outside factors, for the unpredictable changes of reality can never be controlled.

The solution is to find a source of happiness beyond pleasure, since pleasure seeking can never be made independent of outside stimulus. As long as love is pleasure, its end—a sad tapering off into indifference and inertia—is predictable. Recently this argument has gained support from an unexpected quarter. Biochemical research has isolated certain brain chemicals associated with pleasure, particularly the neurotransmitter serotonin. A high level of serotonin is typical of someone who feels a sense of well-being; insufficient levels of serotonin have long been correlated with depression. Related studies have isolated the left frontal lobes of the cortex as a site of increased activity whenever someone feels happy.

The obvious conclusion is that stimulus to the brain is the same as happiness. Unfortunately, this is not accurate, because stimulus wears out. Over time our responses weaken if the same stimulus keeps getting repeated. The taste that was once so sweet grows stale and cloying; the face that once enchanted becomes ordinary; the most exciting vision becomes just part of the scenery.

It is all-important to found our happiness upon a basis that doesn't change. Compared with pleasure, love is abstract. If you took away the pleasant feelings associated with it, most people would be hard-pressed to define the experience of love. But love has a power to heal, to reveal divine essence, to restore faith in one's own Being, to bring harmony to all levels of existence—and all these effects lie far beyond feelings. They are tangible results based on spirit.

In our society the more tangible something is, the more likely we are to have faith in it. Fortunately, for all that love is abstract, scientific research confirms that it is as dramatic and potent as medicine, both when it is present and when it is withdrawn.

Love aids recovery. Studies conducted in hospital cardiac units have demonstrated that male patients who respond positively to the question "Do you feel loved?" are more likely to recover than those who do not, and the correlation between recovery and this response is higher than that for any other category, including previous physical status. In other words, an unloved man in good physical condition afflicted with a mild heart attack may recover more poorly than another man with a severe heart attack who feels loved. For residents of retirement homes, having a pet to love (or even a plant to tend to every day) reduces disease and depression. Old people perceive having an object of love as restoring their purpose in life.

Love promotes growth. Very young children from abusive homes may exhibit a condition of retarded or severely stunted growth known as psychosocial dwarfism. Besides being small and underweight for their age, such children frequently manifest underdeveloped emotions and learning skills. Rapid reversal of this condition can often occur, however, as soon as a loving environment is provided.

Love provides homeostatic balance. No one has definitively proven that feeling loved lowers blood pressure or prevents cancer and heart disease, although it is well documented that negative conditions associated with lack of love, such as chronic anger or depression, put people at much higher risk for all types of disease.

One indication of love's ability to bring the body into balance was provided by a study in which subjects were asked to watch a film about Mother Teresa as she went about her work in India. In the film she embraces children in terribly wasted conditions, usually children afflicted with leprosy. Just the sight of this loving act raised certain chemical indicators of enhanced immune responses. This dramatic effect occurred even if the viewer did not agree with Mother Teresa's vocation—it was not, in other words, a matter of subjectively feeling good. According to folk wisdom, falling in love is the best way not to catch colds in the winter, indicating that the immune benefits of love were recognized long before medical research came along to validate them.

Finally, a breakthrough study from Stanford on recovery from breast cancer indicated that women who were in advanced stages of the disease lived longer if they participated in group therapy sessions once a week, as compared with those who received only normal courses of chemical and surgical treatment. There were no intensive psychological techniques applied here—the group shared their feelings and supported one another in their struggle against cancer. These simple acts of love were provably effective, yet the study underscores how meager one hour of therapy a week really is. Could love on a more intensive scale provide even more healing?

The answer to this question does not await more medical study; it can be verified by each of us in our own lives. *Healing* is a broad term; being connected to both *whole* and *holy,* it can be defined spiritually as a return to the state of unity. Love is not separate from anything in life; it is not divided into moments of love or levels of love or amounts or absence of love. These are our relative terms, our mere glimpses of a force that remains intact and whole. On the spiritual path, or sadhana, the experience of love brings healing that is not directed to one disease or another but to the state of the whole person; therefore each of us will experience its effects differently.

Because sadhana can sound very lofty and abstract, it's easier for science to look at people who are lonely, depressed, and sick than to investigate subtler workings of the self. But if we look at the following features of people who can live a love story, we see how far they have evolved beyond the norm.

*They have learned to separate their actions from their belief*
*that they are lovable.*

Since we all started out as children who were weaker and less powerful than adults, it was only natural for us to try to act in such a way that we wouldn't be hurt. Being hurt is usually a matter of power. The powerless are in no position to offend or antagonize the powerful. This reality was brought home to us on the playground a long time ago, and its holdover habit is trying to be nice. Being nice, we expect niceness in return. By placating someone who threatens us, we hope to ward off aggression. In the name of not being hurt we stay in a defensive posture.

People who base their lives upon love, though, have taught themselves to separate this whole pattern of behavior from love. Love doesn't come from placating potential threats. Being nice all the time won't cause others to love you; when they are stated in black and white this way, most of us would agree with these assertions. Yet the imprint of the past is deep, and unconsciously we still act like powerless children. Learning to grow out of this pattern is a common trait of people who live their own love stories.

*They can give on all levels.*

It has become a truism that to receive love we must give love. This reciprocal action keeps the flow of love alive. Without it love would stagnate. Learning to give runs contrary to some very deep conditioning that we all carry around inside, however. We have all learned to hold on to a good thing. Letting go of anything precious is hard. Loving people have taught themselves that holding on is possessiveness. Anyone who has ever been trapped in a possessive relationship knows its smothering effect. It isn't love when another person cannot give you the space to live your own life.

Giving space isn't simple. You must be willing to allow another person their whole being. You must give permission for someone else's ideas, feelings, reactions, and will to be expressed freely. People who have taught themselves to give on all levels have discovered a critical ingredient of living their love stories.

*They don't expect anything in return for being good.*

We all make a connection between love and goodness. Attraction is based on the assumption that another person has something good to bring into your life. Our definition of this goodness may be shallow or deep. Some men will always believe that a woman is good as long as she is beautiful and compliant. Some women will overlook a dozen things about a man that might spell disaster in a relationship as long as he is dependable and brings in a good income. It takes inner growth to appreciate goodness as a deeper value.

Ultimately people are good because of who they are; goodness is a quality of being. Once we have made this discovery, we stop measuring people by their achievements. We expect goodness as part of their essence, and of ours. When this happens, we no longer expect a reward for doing good. We no longer bestow love when people are good to us and withdraw it when they are bad. Instead love becomes a constant in our lives. It just is. People who have reached this stage are in true possession of their love stories.

*They don't judge or live in fear of judgment.*

Judgment is whatever tells you that there is something wrong with yourself or someone else. Because we all have secrets, we all have some tendency to live in fear of judgment. A voice inside warns us that other people will judge our transgressions as harshly as we do. This self-condemnation has another face—to make ourselves feel safer from being judged, we look for faults in others first. Loving people have taught themselves the falseness of this process. You will never feel better about yourself by making others look worse. Engaging in the habit of criticism only postpones the day when your own secret judgments come to light. Bringing to light whatever you think is wrong about yourself is the only way to diffuse guilt and shame. In reality there is nothing wrong with you or anyone else: this is what the voice of love truly says. Inner growth consists of learning to hear this voice and heed it, a process essential to living your own love story.

*They do not expect others to make them feel loved.*

Love is experienced in relationship. Without someone to love you, the feelings of love—the warmth in a mother's heart, the gladness of friendship, the excitement of intimacy—have no stimulus. That is why the commonest image for being unloved is being alone. When you are alone, there seems to be no relationship. People who find themselves alone rarely feel any incentive to explore love. They await contact with another person or run out to seek it. Thus we become dependent on other people to make us feel totally and permanently loved.

This expectation will, however, always be defeated, and although we blame those who failed to respond to us, who responded but then left, who stayed but then changed their minds, none of them is finally the cause of our problem. The cause is our inability to develop an unshakeable relationship with ourselves. The Self is the source of love. People who live their own love stories have learned this lesson above all.

# In the Absence of Love

The absence of love is as devastating as its presence is beneficial. We will have to assume, unfortunately, that most people are not living a love story right now. Even those who say they are the most deeply in love may be deluding themselves, at least in part. The word *love* applies to so many situations—from intimate affection to abuse, from dependency to control, from lust to ecstasy—that asking if someone feels loved is unreliable.

Lack of love is less elusive, however, so we can more reliably describe what that state feels like. The following are common features of people who are not living their love stories.

*They feel numb and traumatized.*

Once it has grown to fullness, a love based on spirit has no fear of being wounded. Imperfect forms of love are much more vulnerable. Almost everyone has asked for love and received rejection instead. We have taken our frail self-images into situations where they got battered, where hope died and our worst imaginings came true. The effect of rejection, failure, humiliation, and other traumas is to numb one's feelings. Love requires sensitivity. It must have openness. Whatever has numbed you makes it much harder for you to feel love. Therefore people who are numb at the emotional level cannot live their love stories.

*They feel valued for what they do, not for who they are.*

To value yourself is to love yourself. It is really from here that your love for others comes. Value is like currency you can draw from a bank account—if you value yourself a great deal, you actually have something to give to others. If you do not value yourself, you have nothing to draw upon. So what is there to value? If you look at yourself and ask, "What would another person love about me?" the only enduring answer is "Myself." The only people who can give this answer put a value on who they are, not what they do.

Everyone's list of accomplishments is finite. Our good deeds end somewhere. The things about us that society approves of are often outweighed in our own minds by blemishes best kept out of other people's sight. If we value ourselves by what we do—by accomplishments, good deeds, social acceptance—the scope of our love gets limited. People who value themselves almost entirely for what they do will not have love stories of their own.

*They live on distorted beliefs.*

The love you have in your life can only be as valuable as you perceive it to be, and the key to perception is belief. There are no neutral encounters. We always see others in the light of our beliefs; we always feel seen in the light of their beliefs. I've known people who walk into a room full of strangers and believe that a wave of hostility greets them. Other people walk into a room and immediately feel welcome. The difference is entirely one of perception, since this judgment comes before any external evidence. I would say that the first people believe they are not wanted in this world while the other group believe they are.

Any belief that attacks our ability to value ourselves is a distortion. In essence the Self is of highest value; it deserves love without exception. People who cannot live their love stories harbor distorted beliefs that disguise the reality of their infinite worth.

# The Path

*They have failed at love and are too tired to try again.*

When you are faced with a losing enterprise, it's only natural to give up eventually. When we were younger all of us could pursue love with a certain amount of hope and optimism, backed by energy, and it takes energy to carry out any passion. For some people the energy has run out. They say they have no time for love. They feel they do not need it in their lives. What they are actually experiencing is lack of energy, the loss of enthusiasm that follows repeated failure.

But energy is a self-renewing commodity. Like water from a spring, its flow isn't diminished by how much you take away. People who cannot live their love stories have not found a way to renew their energy, to tap into their source of passion.

These various factors don't all apply to any one person. Some of them apply in some degree to all of us. But we can certainly perceive some common underlying causes at work—ignorance of the path to love, how to enter it, how to walk it, even what it is.

Our materialistic worldview has reduced love to a haphazard flow of hormones coupled to psychological fantasies. The spiritual truth is very different. Once the walls fall down we discover that our real problem is that there is *too much* love around us, not too little. Love is eternal and unbounded; it is only we who take tiny sips from its infinite ocean. Rumi states this most natural and yet most secret of mysteries with utter simplicity:

> I look in your inmost self and see the universe not yet created.

The mystery of love hasn't changed across the centuries, we have only fallen short of it. Whenever a person's heart dries up, it may appear that love has dried up. In fact, that person has built a boundary to shut out a force that is always at flood tide. To exist within love's full, unbridled power is terrifying unless you have walked the path to love in complete devotion to the very end.

# LOVING PRACTICE

## Purifying the Heart

You are not going to follow a path that doesn't feel natural for very long, nor will it bring the growth you need, however well intentioned you are. There is a center in the body where love and spirit are joined, and that center is the heart. It is your heart that aches or swells with love, that feels compassion and trust, that seems empty or full. Within the heart is a subtler center that experiences spirit, but spirit is not felt as an emotion or physical sensation. How, then, can you contact it? According to spiritual masters, spirit is experienced first as the absence of what is *not* spirit.

In India this is described as *Netti, netti,* which means, "Not this, not that." Spirit is not caused; it is not bound by time and space; it is not a sensation that can be seen, touched, heard, tasted, or smelled. This may seem like a baffling way to define something, but imagine that you had never seen the color white, that the whole world consisted of red, green, blue, and all the other hues. Then one day a master came to you with a black shirt and said, "If you wash this enough times, you will see that it is white." If you ask to see white before you wash the shirt, what you ask is impossible. Black is the sum of all colors, and only if you wash them all away will white appear.

In the same way your present life is one of sensations, not just colors but all the stimulus that comes through the senses. Some of these sensations may be very pleasurable, but none of them is adequate to tell you what spirit is. Spirit lies beneath the layers of sensations. To experience it you must go to the heart and meditate upon it until everything that obscures spirit is cleansed.

The purpose of the following exercise is to give you the experience of making your heart pure enough to witness spirit. *Pure* here doesn't mean good and virtuous; it means free from impurity, with no value judgment intended. In the words of William Blake, we are cleansing the doors of perception.

### MEDITATING ON THE HEART

Sit comfortably in a quiet room by yourself, choosing a time when you feel settled and unhurried. Early morning is best, since your mind will be alert and fresh; try to avoid late evening, when your awareness is preparing for sleep. Close your eyes and focus your attention on the middle of your chest, where your heart is. (The fact that the physical heart is off to the left is irrelevant here—the spiritual heart center lies directly behind your breastbone.)

Be aware of your heart as a space. Don't try to hear your heartbeat or any other sound you think a heart makes as it pumps blood. The heart center you want to find is a point of awareness where feelings enter. In its pure form it is empty, pervaded by weightlessness, absence of care, peace, and a subtle light. This light may appear as white, gold, pale pink, or blue. But again, don't strain to find a light of any kind. You are not trying to sense the purity of the heart center right now; all you need to feel is whatever is there.

Letting your attention rest easily there, breathe gently and sense your breath going into your heart center. Here you may want to visualize a soft pastel light, or a coolness pervading the chest. Let the breath go in and out, and as it does, ask your heart to speak to you. Don't phrase this as an order; just have the faint intention that you want your heart to express itself.

For the next five or ten minutes, sit and listen. Your heart will begin to release emotions, memories, wishes, fears, and dreams long stored there, and as it does, you will find yourself paying attention.

You may almost immediately get a flash of strong emotion, positive or negative, or a forgotten memory. Your breathing might change. You might gasp or sigh. Let the experience be what it will be. If you daydream or drift off into sleep, don't worry. Just bring your attention back to your heart center. Whether it speaks to you in sadness or fear, delight or pleasure, its message is equally beneficial.

*Paying attention to your heart is the object of this meditation.*

You will notice as you continue this exercise that three things are naturally coming together: meditation, purification, and attention. You are learning to be with your heart in order to heed its spiritual meaning—this is meditation. You are letting repressed material come up to be released—this is purification. You are listening to your heart without judgment or manipulation—this is attention.

Because this process is like washing a shirt to reveal its whiteness, don't be disturbed if strong negative emotions or even physical discomfort starts to appear. Tell yourself that these sensations are leaving; just bid them to go easily and comfortably. If voices of fear, anger, or doubt start to speak, bid them to leave as easily as they want to. (In the case of persistent chest pain, particularly if heart disease is present in your family, you should naturally consult your physician.)

After some days or weeks of practicing this meditation, you will know whether you want to make it a permanent part of your daily routine. I believe that putting attention on the heart is valuable as an addition to any spiritual program; to live from the center of spirit is a constant goal for anyone on the path.

As you progress in the practice, you will begin to notice that sensations, thoughts, memories, daydreams, and random physical manifestations start to decrease. The heart center will slowly reveal itself as it really is: silence, peace, a warm glow, or subtle light. Even if these glimpses are only fleeting, you will find that things are starting to change for you outside meditation. You will start to walk with a more buoyant step. At unexpected moments you will feel a swelling sensation in your chest; you may want to take deep, satisfying breaths. Flashes of elation and well-being may sweep over you at odd times.

All these are signs that the contraction most people hold around their heart center is releasing its grip. The heart center is meant to feel open and relaxed. Before you can receive any profound spiritual insights, this openness must exist. Contraction, fear, tightness all keep spirit from entering you. In truth, spirit doesn't enter, since it is always there. But making contact with it is like being penetrated with light and insight; this is what we call the flow of love.

Love and spirit are forming a connection every time you meditate on the heart, starting with the first time. Advanced meditation deepens this experience and makes it more conscious. As you continue this practice, you will find it easier and easier to go to your heart for counsel and wisdom, or simply to feel that you are loved. You do not have to speak to your heart in words; your heart doesn't have to speak to you in words. The language of spirit comes to us as silent assurance, self-acceptance, patience, an appreciation of simply being. As these qualities develop you are maturing in your experience of the heart center.

# In Our Lives

## "Who Will Rescue Me?"

Her name was Nina. On the surface she presented herself as someone in supreme control of her life. She was an intelligent, gifted woman who had independent financial means and used them in a socially conscious way. Privately she was intensely spiritual. I would regularly get late-night calls when Nina couldn't wait to talk about some new discovery that had excited her in her voracious reading of scriptures, masters, and "messages" of every sort. I knew Nina from earlier days in Boston when she sat on our hospital board, and I had attended her latest wedding early this year.

It took place on a mountainside in Oregon facing a spectacular Pacific sunset. The vows exchanged between the bride and groom were unconventional; in addition to elements drawn from the familiar Christian service, the vows contained a Buddhist prayer and New Age verses about soul mates finding each other across the universe. The joy in the air could be felt like a warm, nourishing rain from the twilit skies.

For Nina this ceremony marked a huge personal milestone. "I'm going to do it right this time," she had declared. At forty-five Nina had already been married and raised two grown children. Her divorce had been the result of outgrowing her old self-image, which was much more conventional than spiritual. "I lived the way my mother taught me—don't think about yourself, make your husband and children happy. If your love is selfless enough, things will take care of themselves," she said.

But after nineteen years Nina didn't feel taken care of. Her love had supported other people but not herself. She decided to find self-improvement on her own. Therapy, meditation retreats, and women's groups quickly followed. When her husband resisted these changes, Nina felt fearful but determined. The door to self-exploration was open, and she wanted her relationships to mirror the new person she was trying to become.

She explained, "If my first husband insisted on keeping me in a box that I didn't want to be in, then he wasn't the person who loved me the most. It had taken me a long time, but that was what I wanted out of marriage, to be with a person who could accept me and allow me to grow. That's my idea of someone who loves me the most." Nina felt she had found such a mate in Gregory; after a whirlwind romance that began through having the same therapist in Los Angeles, Nina rushed into marriage a few months after her divorce.

Ten months later I saw her at a reception and asked, "How's Gregory?"

Nina's eyes grew vague. "Oh, we're having problems. We both thought it might be good to have some time apart. I don't know— things happened." Her voice drifted off; she looked exhausted. I hardly recognized the woman who had placed such high hopes on her marriage.

Nina later confided that although Gregory wasn't dominant or demanding like her first husband, she found herself getting angry at him and distrusting his motives in marrying her; they were both spiritual, but the soul love she had expected wasn't there. One thing Nina said was extremely telling: "Do you want to know something?

Every morning when I wake up, I repeat the same question to myself: 'Who will rescue me?' "

"Who do you think will?" I asked.

She shrugged. "Maybe nobody, I don't know."

I knew Nina well enough to be sure that she doesn't see herself as merely a victim or a damsel in distress. There was a deeper reason why this question was coming up. Nina was expressing the fundamental, haunting fear of aloneness. "Who will rescue me?" means, "Am I going to survive on my own?" This fear bespeaks our tremendous need for security, a need so dominant that it often blocks the insight, courage, and freedom we really need but don't know how to find.

When we had time alone I laid this out for Nina, telling her that I thought the speed of her courtship and subsequent decision to marry Gregory said a lot about her insecurity after her divorce.

"When we set out on a spiritual path, we set out on a solitary journey, yet pulling against this is all the old conditioning that tells us, particularly women, that it isn't safe to go it alone, that we can't make it without outside support. In other words, commitment to yourself collides with your belief in commitment to a mate. Society is changing, and independence for both sexes is more accepted than before, yet that doesn't change the feeling of aloneness that hits you when you break away from old conventions, old models, old social standards."

"Then I have to choose either marriage or being by myself?" Nina asked.

"No," I answered, "that's just fear talking. Your love for Gregory can be the starting point for finding yourself; the two aren't incompatible."

Spirituality begins with a vision, but reality doesn't fit that vision. The path is what brings them together. Most people who want to experience inner growth begin, as Nina did, by reading in the vast inspirational literature. They become discontented with the distance between their own lives and the enlightened existence they discover in their reading; they start to make a break. Inevitably there turn out to be people—like Nina's first husband or parents or old friends—who don't fit the spiritual vision. Yet after the break nothing seems to really change. The haunting insecurity and loneliness, the sense of confusion and conflict, are still there.

But instead of feeling let down by this "failure," you need to realize that all spiritual work is done by yourself, with yourself, and for yourself. No one "out there" can take responsibility. It is all right to be aware of a distance between vision and reality, because that is what it feels like to be on the path. If you had no gaps to close, you wouldn't need a path.

We all step onto the path to love out of need, but at a certain point need can be destructive, because it is born of lack and fear. Need must be balanced with two other ingredients—willingness to be transformed and support in that transformation.

It isn't easy to have all these requirements met, and it's nearly impossible if you don't know of their existence. A highly motivated woman like Nina would find it particularly difficult to expose her vulnerability, to express need directly. Her willingness to change seemed genuine, since that was the motivation behind her divorce, but was this willingness really deep? In choosing Gregory, who had much experience of spiritual matters, she found the opposite of her first husband, but perhaps Gregory saw too clearly into her insecurities. Finally, support depends upon being able to receive it when it is offered, and it wasn't clear that Nina was entirely open to sharing herself with a man whom she had known for only a few months before they began to live together.

Need, willingness, and support. All of these are necessary if one is to step onto the path to love. They serve as signals to spirit that you are ready to depart from traditional ways of living, for the old modes can't be converted to new ones.

I told Nina that there was a deeper meaning to her question "Who will rescue me?" She was expressing an intuition that she was going to be rescued. But not by a man—it was her own spirit that was summoning her onto the path.

I asked Nina to practice meditating on her heart, and this is what she said she felt: gasps and moments of ragged breathing, occasional sobs followed by deep, relaxed sighs, twinges of chest pain, tightness in her neck and abdomen, restless urges to stop meditating and jump out of her chair. When asked what was happening mentally, she reported flashes of old memories, bursts of sadness, fantasies, obsessive repetition of daily worries, and some fleeting moments of silence.

This is very typical of a person newly opening up to spirit—a lot of purification was going on as the mind body system began to release its old energies. Nina's transformation, like everything placed in the hands of spirit, promised to be tremendously beautiful. For the time being, however, she was too caught up in her confusions to see this.

At one point in our conversation, Nina was startled by a comment I made. "If you don't mind me saying so, I like you this way," I said.

"What? In a mess?" she rejoined.

"First of all, I don't think you're in a mess. You're in ferment, and there's a big difference. Your confusion has made you open."

"You mean it's turned my life upside down," she corrected.

"And what's wrong with that? We can all be wounded, every one of us. The people who try to deny this have to live inside a shell of denial. That's not what you want."

She suddenly looked tired. "I just want to be happy."

"That's what everyone wants, but you're aiming much higher," I said. "You want to be real. And you're willing to face what it takes to get there. That's how your spirit is expressing itself right now."

Her mood broke, and she gave me a wan smile. "Having a warm body next to me would help."

There's nothing obviously "spiritual" about Nina's situation, but in fact the path to love beckons most strongly when old behaviors, beliefs, and approaches no longer work. Ferment, restlessness, and discontent always mark the beginning of the path.

Before we parted Nina and I embraced. "You don't feel loved right now," I said, "and you doubt whether you are lovable. You feel instead that you have failed or been let down. Allow these feelings to be what they are; don't try to run away from them. But know that the real issue lies somewhere else—you are trapped in a definition of love that is far too limited. Expand your definition, allow your conception of love to go beyond your emotional needs, and your whole perspective will change. You won't see failure and defeat. Far from it—you'll see perfection. At every moment, from the second you were conceived in the womb, your life has been about love. Your existence is an expression of love, the only real expression it can have. Everything else is an illusion."

# 3

# THE SPIRIT OF
# ROMANCE

— ✿ —

In our culture we are not taught to see falling in love as a spiritual event, yet for centuries that was the accepted interpretation. When the question "Where does love come from?" was asked, the universal answer was God. According to the New Testament,

> He that loveth not knoweth not God; for God is love.

The lives of saints of every religion have demonstrated love in its spiritual dimension; at the same time the humblest person who fell in love also realized he was treading on sacred ground. Over the centuries, particularly in the West, the divine connection was lost, however, and romantic love became a more earthly matter, more centered in the entrancing charms of another individual ("How do I love thee, let me count the ways").

In spiritual terms falling in love is an opening, an opportunity to step into the timeless and stay there, to learn the ways of spirit and bring them down to earth. All openings are temporary—this is not a limitation specific to falling in love. The real question is, What should we do with the opening? The highest spiritual qualities—those of truth, faith, trust, and compassion—grow from the tiniest seeds of daily experience. Their first sproutings are exceedingly vulnerable, and there is no guarantee they will not wither and die. How can we tend this fragile opening of the heart, nurture it until it develops into more substantial stages of growth?

To do that we must examine romance, the first stage in love's journey, as part of a timeless cycle that brings greater and greater knowledge of spiritual reality. The insights of this first stage are, naturally enough, those relating to a new birth:

*Love knows that you exist and cares for your existence.*

*Timeless spirit can touch you in this world of time.*

*With a new birth of the heart, you will see a new world.*

*Love is never old but renews itself with every lover.*

*Flesh and spirit can share in the same delights.*

*All people are innocent in the light of love.*

When you fall in love these insights come to you like fresh water, yet they are as ancient as the path to love itself. The sensation of romantic love is so overwhelming that it is easy to neglect the value of these insights; they are among the most joyous that anyone can experience here on earth. For lovers inner growth begins in a state of rapture.

There are four distinct phases of romance. Although not everyone can expect to experience them exactly the same way, all four naturally emerge once your feelings for someone else go beyond friendship to passionate attachment. The four phases are

Attraction

Infatuation

Courtship

Intimacy

Attraction begins when one person picks out, through means usually totally unknown and unconscious, another person to be smitten by. Infatuation, in which the beloved becomes all-desirable and all-enveloping, soon follows. In the depths of infatuation the lover's fantasy life can become both wild and extreme. If there are no insurmountable barriers, the phase of courtship will arrive next. The beloved is wooed to create the same attraction the lover so overwhelmingly feels.

If the courtship is successful, intimacy follows. The underlying sexual excitement that plays such a strong part in romance, and that at first is restrained by the outlet of fantasy, is now allowed fulfillment. Through intimacy the union of two people begins to be played out in the real world rather than within an isolated psyche. Reality dawns as the lovers' rosy images get tested against a real person. For better or worse, there is an unmasking of fantasy, and the way is cleared for the next stage of love's journey, relationship.

These four phases of romance occur in a natural, linear sequence, but at the same time they come full circle. For a time lover and beloved are exempted from everyday reality; extraordinary states of emotion and attraction place them on a privileged plane. Once fantasy is unmasked, either the lovers will find themselves fallen back to earth or they will have learned from their experience and will be ready to integrate it into love's further growth.

Although it happens spontaneously, falling in love isn't accidental—there are no accidents in the spiritual life, only patterns we haven't yet recognized.

*All love is based on the search for spirit.*

This is the first major insight to be found in romantic love—it really isn't about two people who have fallen madly for each other; it is about two people seeing spirit in each other.

One expression of this idea comes from ancient India; here the mythic king Yajnavalkya is speaking about love to his queen:

> Truly, it is not for the sake of the husband that the husband is dear, but for the sake of the Self.
>
> And it is not for the sake of the wife that the wife is dear, but for the sake of the Self.
>
> And it is not for the sake of the sons that the sons are dear, but for the sake of the Self.
>
> Indeed, my beloved, it is the Self that should be seen, the Self that should be heard, the Self that should be reflected upon, and the Self that should be known.

This passage from the "great forest teaching" *(Brihadaranyaka Upanishad)* dates from thousands of years ago. If what it proclaims is true, then falling in love is undeniably an act of the soul. Falling in love drives you to passionate merging with your beloved, but the deeper passion is for the Self, the source of all love.

# THE SECRET OF ATTRACTION

Any creature capable of reproducing with another of its kind must feel attraction, but humans are unique in that we can see *meaning* in our attraction. Hence there is a huge difference between falling in love unconsciously, as if struck by a bolt of lightning, and consciously embracing love's gift with full knowledge that this is what your soul craves, what you live for, what you will put foremost in your life.

In ancient India the ecstasy of love was called *Ananda,* or bliss consciousness. The ancient seers held that humans are meant to partake of this ananda at all times. As I noted before, one famous verse of the Vedas declares of humans, "In bliss they were conceived, in bliss they live, to bliss they will return." Ananda is much more than pleasure, even the most intense erotic pleasure. It is one-third of the formula for the spirit's true nature, described by the Vedas as *Sat Chit Ananda,* or eternal bliss consciousness.

As we shall see, the path to love ends with the full realization of this simple phrase. *Sat* is eternal truth upholding everything in existence; when sat is fully established, there is no evil or suffering because nothing is separate from unity. *Chit* is the consciousness of that unity; it is the fullness of peace that has no possibility of being disturbed by fear. *Ananda* is the ultimate joy of being in this awareness; it is the unchanging bliss that all glimpses of ecstasy aim to become. The path of love carries us to full knowledge of all three aspects without doubts. But the one we taste most often here on earth is the last—ananda—in the joy of falling in love.

> *Romance is set apart from all other forms of love by the intensity of bliss.*

Two people who fall under each other's spell experience a revolution in their deepest beings from the sudden discovery that bliss has dawned. Spiritual masters tell us that we were born in bliss, but this condition gets obscured by the chaotic activity of everyday life. Below the chaos, however, we are trying to find ananda again; all lesser joys are tiny drops, while ananda is the ocean.

The insights that apply to this phase grow from our yearning to find bliss:

> *Bliss is natural to life, but once we cover it over, we must search for it in others.*
>
> *The pain of yearning is a mask for the ecstasy of bliss.*
>
> *Bliss is not a feeling but a state of being.*
>
> *In the state of bliss, everything is loved.*

Our hunger to return to bliss is one reason why falling in love is never accidental. We all have the subconscious knowledge of what love can do to the psyche. An isolated person, full of frustration and loneliness, is suddenly transformed, made complete beyond the power of reason to explain. In place of anxiousness and doubt there is ecstasy. According to the New Testament,

> There is no fear in love; but perfect love casteth out fear.

This blissful sense of being in a place of peace and safety lasts through the beginning stages of romance, despite the emotional ups and downs that inevitably follow.

Yet ananda is often the last thing we think we will find, because before we fall in love there is an anxious period of intense longing. This state is the negative of romance, yet it is also its true beginning, for without separation and yearning, there could be no attraction. To find bliss we have to begin where bliss is not. In our society this is not a hard place to locate.

## THE ANXIOUS SEARCH

Attraction depends upon finding someone to love or having that someone find you, and here the difficulties begin. If nothing is more exalted than falling in love, then nothing seems to arouse more fearfulness. A constant, anxious search for relationship seems to haunt our whole society. We are inundated with images of romantic attraction, yet ironically the real thing seems very elusive, and the more heavily our television and movies pile on the seductive charm, the more tenuously people appear to understand what love actually is.

The sensation of falling in love is not hard to describe. It has been compared to a thousand delights, from the sweetness of honey to the fragrance of a rose. Its images are legion, and we are surrounded by them, as if total immersion will somehow resolve our underlying insecurity. When romance actually dawns, however, it is more intoxicating than any packaged image, because romance distills love and desire, eager longing and tender suffering, the joy of a single moment's touch and the agony of a single moment's separation.

All this we know, yet knowledge has done little to dispel the anxious feeling that love is never going to arrive, that we are not quite right in some way and therefore do not deserve this astonishing gift called falling in love. As most of us go about it, our search for love is driven by two potent psychological forces: a fantasy of ideal romance and a fear that we will miss out and never be loved at all.

Both these drives are self-defeating, although in different ways. If you carry around an idealized fantasy of what love should be like, you will miss the real thing when it crosses your path. Real love begins with everyday interactions that hold the seed of promise, not with full-blown ecstasy. The seed is easy to overlook, and nothing blinds us to it more than fixed mental images.

In much the same way, if you go around in a state of anxiety about whether someone will pick you out to love, you will never make yourself attractive to anyone, for nothing kills romance quicker than fear. To strive to be attractive is just another form of desperation, which others see no matter how hard you struggle to disguise it. So strong is our social conditioning, however, that billions more dollars are spent on cosmetics, fashion, and plastic surgery than on psycho-therapy, for example, despite the fact that working on their neuroses would make most people much more attractive than a svelte figure or designer clothes.

Despite their self-defeating nature, these two motivations—fantasy and fear—are what most of us fall back on when we search for love. Prompted by them, men and women approach romance with behaviors that can never bring about what they hope to achieve. These tactics all grow out of listening to an inner voice that obsesses about love and directs our search even though the voice itself is quite loveless. Most of these futile behaviors will sound extremely familiar:

- ➤ We constantly compare ourselves with an ideal that we can never live up to. The loveless inner voice drives us by saying, "You aren't good enough—thin enough, pretty enough, happy enough, secure enough."
- ➤ We look for approval in others. This behavior basically projects our inner dissatisfaction with ourselves in the hope that some outside authority will lift it from our souls. Here the loveless inner voice is saying, "Don't make a move until the right person comes along." (The right person in this

THE PATH to LOVE

case is some fairy-tale character who will tap the ugly duckling and turn it into a swan.) Being an impossible fiction, that right person never arrives.

➤ We assume that falling in love is totally magical, a stroke from the blue that will come at random, usually when least expected. Many people wait passively for this magic to appear. Although masked as hope, this passivity is really a form of hopelessness, for the inner loveless voice is saying, "There's nothing you can do but wait to see if someone loves you." The underlying belief here is that we cannot possibly deserve love—not the passionate, fulfilling love of our dreams. The hope that someone will reach out to us and bestow love is a surrender of our ability to create our own lives.

➤ Finally, we rely on love to remove the obstacles that keep it away. All sorts of unloving behaviors are allowed to persist with the attitude that we will become affectionate, open, trusting, and intimate only by a touch of love's magic wand. The inner loveless voice keeps us in total inertia by saying, "It doesn't matter how you treat all these people. After all, they don't love you, and when the ideal person comes along, these people will matter even less." The underlying belief in this case is that we can pick and choose whom to love, leaving the rejected in a limbo of indifference.

Can we find another way to approach romance, without fantasy and fear, without listening to the fearful voice inside ourselves that finds a way to keep love at a distance?

## "TO LOVE, BE LOVABLE"

To begin with, we can't keep confining romance to an emotional state; we must redefine it as a surrender to the mystery of our own spirit—sat chit ananda—for beneath the turbulence of emotion that is what romance is. It is a state in which your primary relationship is not with your beloved but with your Self. Romance therefore begins when you can show your soul to another person.

The secret to being attractive, if one consults the past record of human experience, is remarkably simple. It is summarized in an aphorism from the Latin poet Ovid, who said, "To love, be lovable." A lovable person is someone who is natural, easy with himself or herself, radiating the simple, unaffected humanity that makes anyone truly attractive.

Sometimes, however, the simplest solutions are the most difficult to achieve. People find themselves caught up in the anxious search for love precisely because they don't feel lovable. The very condition that would make for romance is absent. It is sad to say, but many of us have never felt lovable, even in childhood, when we had the fewest defenses against love and therefore could approach it with the most spontaneous innocence. A child who does not easily ask for affection and attention, who does not blossom when these are supplied, or who lives with her or his appeals unanswered, has been deprived of the very essence of childhood. Even for those of us who were loved adequately as children and therefore are in touch with our lovableness, bringing it forth is incredibly difficult in the current social climate.

Being lovable isn't a superficial quality; it is a quality of spirit. Ananda cannot be destroyed, only covered over. In the end, if you can see yourself as spirit, it won't matter what conditioning has occurred in the past, whether you were fortunate enough to be raised with loving values or so unfortunate that you were discouraged and made to feel ugly and worthless. Remember, in our inmost being, we are all completely lovable because spirit *is* love. Beyond what anyone can make you think or feel about yourself, your unconditioned spirit stands, shining with a love nothing can tarnish.

If being lovable really is the secret to attraction, then there is no need for anxious searching, because your own being, which can never be lost, doesn't have to be found. The whole futile process of making yourself attractive to others, of constantly waiting for someone else's response, of desperately comparing yourself with an ideal image can come to an end. The only requirement is a shift in perception, for those who cannot find love perceive themselves as not being lovable. This is not true, but they make it seem true by linking their perception to a powerful system of beliefs.

*What creates romance is the ability to see yourself as lovable.*

This shift in perception happens not by changing who you are but by seeing who you are and then shining it forth. If you were able to exhibit the full grandeur of your being, your whole life would be a romance, one long love story dedicated to ecstasy and joy. Rumi puts it elegantly when he declares,

> By God, when you see your beauty
> You'll be the idol of yourself.

Nothing is more beautiful than naturalness. It alone contains the mystery and allure that spark romance. Trying to be cosmetically attractive is beside the point, for we are talking here about authenticity.

We all covet images of intensely desirable people, generally actors and models who make their living by appearing to be desirable. In reality, however, they are likely to be extremely insecure about their desirability, since their value is subject to the whims of a public they have never met. Aspiring to these images is aspiring to be something that you are not.

The farther you are from the desired image, the harder you must try to suppress who you really are. The tendency is to make yourself more and more inauthentic, until, if you "succeed" in becoming as desirable as your image, you will have thrown away what is most desirable in yourself—your unique, multifaceted being. This being doesn't live up to any single image, ugly or beautiful, desirable or undesirable, because it expresses the shifting, changing light of life. This light is nothing if not ambiguous. Your being contains shadows and hints of meaning; it is mysterious to the core.

To be authentic, you have to be everything that you are, omitting nothing. Within everyone there is light and shadow, good and evil, love and hate. The play of these opposites is what constantly moves life forward; the river of life expresses itself in all its changes from one opposite to another. If you can truly embrace these opposites within yourself, you will be authentic, and as your self-acceptance expands until there is nothing to be ashamed of, nothing to hide, your life will take on the generosity and warmth that marks every great lover.

*Being desirable means being comfortable with your own ambiguity.*

The ultimate ambiguity that each of us expresses is not that we can be both good and bad, loving and unloving, but that we are spirit and flesh at the same time. Nothing could be more ambiguous than this, or more alluring.

# LOVING PRACTICE

## Accepting Ambiguity

Most of us waste our time trying to become more attractive, particularly by concentrating on the most superficial level of attraction, the physical. Not only is physical beauty temporary, which means that fixating on it will pay decreasing dividends over time, its ideals are never met either.

If you are imprisoned by physical images, you are certain deep down inside that you will never be attractive enough. This certainty leads women to obsessively improve their inevitable weak points through cosmetics and clothing. Although men may trivialize the beauty issue as female vanity, their own huge expenditures on sports cars, designer golf clubs, and power suits is a product of the same insecurity. There is only one way to break out of the self-defeating syndrome of "I'll never look good enough."

*What will really make you attractive is not working on your weak points but embracing them.*

Embracing your weaknesses is the same as accepting yourself, and nothing is more attractive than people who are comfortable with themselves. Weak points do not have to be physical—any trait that you think makes you unattractive falls into this category, including psychological foibles, lack of money or success, low social standing, and past actions you feel must be covered up.

A person who exhibits both positive and negative qualities, strengths and weaknesses, is not flawed but complete. At any given moment our behavior has shadings; it is never a simple matter of black or white. These shadings are what I call the appeal of ambiguity, which the following exercise helps to develop. Approach it as a free-form activity, in keeping with the spirit of ambiguity.

## FILLING IN THE SHADOWS

The purpose of the following exercise is to take any quality you think you possess and demonstrate that you also possess its opposite—and many variations in between. You can perform this exercise in your head, but I recommend pencil and paper.

Write down or think about one particular thing that makes you unattractive to others. It can be physical or psychological, whatever comes first to mind. Let's say it's "I'm too selfish."

Ask yourself if you also have the opposite trait, which is "I'm considerate of other people's needs." Or, if this sounds too altruistic, try "I am not selfish all the time." (This has to be true, since no one can be selfish 100 percent of the time.) Having set this down, notice that being considerate doesn't cancel out being selfish—it adds another shade to the picture. All traits, good and bad, are relative. They can never completely describe who you really are.

*Who you really are is not a collection of parts but a whole. Seeing yourself as whole is the first step toward seeing yourself as truly attractive.*

We are all tempted to pick ourselves apart; it is this act of self-criticism, not the pieces themselves, that makes you feel unattractive.

Now move on to another undesirable quality; this time choose one that is trivial enough that you are ashamed of admitting you even care about it—for example, "My hips are too big."

Now find the opposite of feeling ashamed of this trait, which can be phrased in several ways, such as "Marilyn Monroe had big hips, and she looked beautiful," or "The last time I felt good about myself, I wasn't thinking about my hips," or "Someone who really loves me has assured me that hips are not what matters to him."

These responses work on different levels. If your friends say they don't notice your hips, the issue may become not whether they are right but whether you trust them. By seeing more ambiguity in the situation, you start to grasp how complex and interconnected everything about you is. As you break the grip of your conditioning, challenging your notion of a bad or weak quality by considering its opposite, you free your mind to see the larger picture about yourself.

You can turn this into a very creative exercise. Suppose you write down "I bad-mouth my best friends," a characteristic most of us would find extremely unattractive. The offsetting quality might be "I really do love my best friends." What is the relationship between these opposing traits? Perhaps you aren't comfortable telling your best friend when you are angry or disappointed; perhaps you lash out indiscriminately when you feel bad about yourself; perhaps you want to be liked so much that you criticize your friends to reinforce someone else's opinion.

All these alternatives underscore a single truth: you are only human. When you realize that the same is true of every person you've ever met (as well as every media darling celebrated in our society), you will gain a sense of comfort with both the most attractive people and the least attractive. The closer you come to seeing the appeal in all people, the closer you come to God's perspective.

*Equality is the first step toward acceptance, and acceptance is love.*

Try articulating a few more of your worst qualities, then move on to your good ones. What is most attractive about you? "I have lovely eyes." "I adore my children." "I contribute time to helping cancer patients." Whatever you write down, see if the opposite isn't also present. "My eyes aren't very lovely when I'm jealous or mean." "My children can make me feel like running away." "Sick people depress me so much, I don't care if I ever see another one." Whatever you find in yourself that is nice or good, it is inevitable that the contrary impulse also exists in you. No saint has ever lived who did not blame and hate God in her darkest hour; no lover is so smitten that he has not noticed the allure of another woman.

The final stage of this exercise involves reading the following list:

It is all right to be good and bad.

I like feeling more than one way about the people who are closest to me.

Niceness can have an edge; snideness can be amusing.

My best friend wouldn't be shocked to see me at my worst. My worst enemy would be pleasantly surprised to see me at my best.

Living up to my self-image is more exhausting than I let on.

I'll never be perfect. I can live with that.

An angel is assigned to people who can laugh in the face of misery.

THE PATH *to* LOVE

It's all right to find the villain sexy and the hero boring.
I will trust the next person who tells me I look good.
Letting the demons run can be very educational
  sometimes.
The worst thing anyone says about me contains some truth
  —about them.

You are likely to agree with some of these statements, and a few may seem preposterous or beside the point. Be that as it may, the next time you sit down to do this exercise, look over the list again. You may be surprised at how much more acceptable it seems. Accepting your own ambiguity opens you to the truth that life itself cannot help but be ambiguous, which is what makes it so fascinating.

# In Our Lives

## What's a Little Gray?

When she found a bottle of black hair dye in Alan's drawer, Jeanne passed it off as a touch of middle-aged male vanity. She had always thought of her husband as intensely attractive; in fact, given how much younger he was than she—seven and a half years—Jeanne had been secretly flattered to catch him. Looking in the mirror, she noticed more gray in her hair than he ever had.

Jeanne had found the bottle of dye late at night while looking for aspirin; it was in a drawer she usually didn't open. The next morning she asked Alan about it as he was rushing out the door. He looked surprised and said the dye wasn't his.

Jeanne didn't know whether to believe him or not. This feeling surprised her, since she had always assumed that Alan could be trusted. Jeanne had some time to kill before she went off to her own job—there was no baby to attend to, since the couple, married just three years, had decided not to have children. She found herself cleaning out the clutter in the bathroom cabinets. No more bottles.

Jeanne brought up the incident over lunch with her best friend Cecille, making light of it. Cecille looked worried. "I don't know how to put this, but if I were you, I'd be careful."

"Of what?" Jeanne asked.

"Hasn't it occurred to you that your husband might be having an affair?"

Of course it hadn't. Jeanne flushed scarlet; she didn't like having suspicions planted in her head, but instead of saying so she asked Cecille to elaborate. You can't let yourself go, her best friend warned, not for a minute. From the age of three little boys are taught that when they grow up they will have power; they expect to run things from the time they are in the sandbox. Little girls, by contrast, are trained to be worthy of men with power, which means being beautiful enough to attract them. If she isn't able to hold a man, what power does a woman have? With considerable earnestness Cecille advised Jeanne to buy a hundred-dollar facial and some skimpy lingerie.

Jeanne didn't know what to make of her friend's little speech—a mixture of fascination, doubt, and dread warred inside her. But why would Alan lie about something as trivial as a bottle of hair dye if he wasn't hiding something else? Jeanne decided that buying a sheer nightgown wasn't the worst idea in the world, and when she brought it home her husband looked pleased. He had a lot of work to do that night, however, and the amorous evening she had planned didn't pan out. Alan seemed less than involved when they made love; he fell asleep without saying anything. Jeanne had promised herself that she would never wheedle the words "I love you" from Alan, but that night it was hard to keep the promise.

Jeanne began to feel that Alan probably *was* having an affair, and why shouldn't he? He was hardly aging at all, while she was falling apart. It's always faster with a woman, she mourned, and new nightgowns weren't going to reverse things. Nobody had ever commented to her face about the age disparity between herself and Alan, but Jeanne had no doubt that their friends, especially the women, all remarked about it behind her back. She began to have fantasies about who the other woman was.

The downward spiral would have been swift, but it came to a merciful halt thanks to second-class mail. A week later an identical bottle of hair dye arrived in the mailbox. Jeanne went back to the bathroom drawer—the first bottle also said "free sample" on the back. She now vaguely remembered having pitched it into the drawer without really looking at what it was. Jeanne didn't know whether to laugh or cry.

As I see it, this incident isn't really about how attractive a woman feels. It's about how deserving she feels. We all attach self-worth to outside things. Status, money, a big house, all become in some way a reflection on "me." We also do this with other people. To be attached to someone young and good looking becomes an important part of "me" if I feel I lack those qualities. Any lack we feel can be filled in this way, by projection, but as soon as the connection is broken, projection fails.

"When romantic love is at its height," I told Jeanne, "it's only natural to want to sustain it. Romance is selfish, in that you become absorbed in your feelings. When you fell in love with Alan, his attractiveness—or yours—had nothing to do with the inner experience. Delight in another person, the feeling that you have met a perfect being, is only a reflection of what you have suddenly remembered in yourself."

"But there are beautiful people," Jeanne said.

"Are there people who are not?" I asked. "Setting certain people aside as beautiful is simply image-making, which actually obscures the larger truth that, in the eyes of spirit, no one is excluded from the highest state of perfection. How do you feel when you look at an extremely attractive person?"

"More than one thing," replied Jeanne. "If he was mine, I'd feel proud, but there's also a good deal of insecurity involved—that's no secret now."

"The whole strategy of being beautiful by proxy can never work," I said. "Not only are you living vicariously, which is always fragile at best, but you are not coming from a place of love. Using another person isn't loving; it's treating that person like an object. Objects always wear out, or the joy we take in them fades. More important, using someone as an object forces you to miss his value as a human being."

I asked Jeanne to examine what this incident said about her. She might begin with this lesson: *You are only as attractive as you feel you deserve to be.* Deservedness is the deep issue that beauty hides. Someone who is deserving can be open to love in all its spiritual significance; someone who is not will be limited to love that includes fear, since what you don't deserve can always be taken from you.

"This issue of what you deserve arouses insecurity," I said, "only if you put it in isolated terms. Spiritually, we are all totally deserving because we are all whole. If your being includes everything, how can you deserve one thing less than another? This sense of completeness isn't material. It doesn't consist of being absolutely beautiful, infinitely rich, or impeccably virtuous. The miracle of love is that you can be imperfect and still be completely whole."

This last point isn't easy to grasp. But if you consider how a mother loves her child, it is immediately obvious that the imperfections of the child do not count in her eyes. This isn't blindness but the vision of love. Love is extremely sensitive to weaknesses. It responds by wanting to support and lend strength in any way possible. But there is no judgment in it against weakness or defect. A mother helping her toddler to walk isn't thinking, "If you were competent, you'd be walking on your own by now." She accepts that growth moves by stages and takes it as her joy to nurture each stage. The question is, how can she do this for herself?

Jeanne could have just let her anxiety in this one instance pass—that was always an option—but the beginning of wisdom would be to take this opportunity to learn how to reconsider her insecurity. Every time she thinks, "I'm too old," she should follow it with "That doubt isn't me." Every time she thinks, "Alan is too young for me," she should follow it with "That insecurity isn't me." Every time she thinks, "Another woman is interested in my husband," she should follow it with "That suspicion isn't me." Bringing the issue home to herself instead of projecting it onto an external object will make it easier to face her responsibility for creating all her false beliefs.

"Situations mirror beliefs," I told her. "Removing other people from the picture and bringing every moment of self-doubt back to its real source is the best way to stay focused on the truth."

Having found the truth, Jeanne can begin the inner work of solving her concealed issues. Being an "older woman" has never been entirely comfortable for her, and living in proximity to Alan's nonchalance about their age difference hasn't really helped. "You should make it clear to Alan," I said, "that you need reassurance. He is the right person to ask for this, not your best friend."

Clearly Jeanne desperately wants her husband to say "I love you" at times, yet she forces herself not to ask. She therefore pushes herself further into self-doubt, by forbidding herself to ask for what she wants. This self-denial is a result of shame, an emotion closely connected to deservedness. "You need to realize that asking to be loved is not only not shameful," I said, "it's exactly what one should do to get love. Shame tells us that love is a small, precious commodity that we have to beg for, like Oliver Twist begging for another bowl of soup. But love is abundant, and asking for it only reflects that you already perceive it to be yours."

Whenever Alan says that he loves her, Jeanne also needs to trust his assurance, and if this proves difficult, she should resist the temptation to ask for more reassurance on the spot—it will be more productive to work on how she can learn to trust.

Here the story comes to a parting between psychology and spirituality. In psychological terms Jeanne's lack of self-worth is bound up in dark memories from her past. As a small girl she was imprinted with experiences that told her she wasn't good enough—we all have similarly painful memories. Years later these were transferred to looks, age, and sexual desirability. Jeanne would never accept herself as long as she was attracted to men who she believed were more desirable than she, because any comparison would put her in the shade. Being with Alan was a "solution" born out of past conditioning that had to fall away.

Having gotten this far in her analysis, I told Jeanne that she could open the trapdoor under which many secret hurts and shadowy fears lurk. Confronting secret shame and guilt is a valid psychological approach to her sort of problem. The unanswered question, however, is whether it is possible to release every demon and doubt, every painful memory and negative energy. Few who have attempted such a massive undertaking have succeeded without the aid of spirit.

"I think it's a good idea for you to work through personal issues," I told Jeanne, "but a lasting solution to whether you are deserving or not will only come spiritually. Here's something useful to write down as a reminder:

*"Spirit is always with me. It wants to lift my pain. It does this not by abolishing painful memories but by putting me totally in the present, where the past doesn't exist.*

"The spiritual answer to any problem is immediate," I said. "It's our own perception that is slow to catch on. God's ability to love us is limited only by our ability to receive that love here and now. Since our loved ones represent manifested portions of God in our lives, the same could be said for them. To receive God's love we need only increase our ability to receive the love being reflected back in our intimate relationships."

As for many people, what really lay at the heart of Jeanne's difficulties was a tendency to pre-reject herself. Instead of assuming that she must be imperfect, she could start noticing how her husband really feels. In my experience, if you are getting stuck in negativity, you're likely to assume that other people feel the same way about you, and mostly that's not true. People who really love you keep on loving you, even when you're not loving yourself.

At an unconscious level Jeanne's pre-rejection of herself has kept her on the lookout for the slightest reason that someone else should also reject her. The more accepting others are, the more she believes she has to be vigilant. The hidden belief here is that the more loving her husband is, the smaller the slip needed to destroy that love. In reality, love doesn't work this way. Alan's deepening love for his wife would make him accept and forgive more and more of what she sees as unworthy in herself. Thus the spiritual truth is validated: the love you get is limited only by your ability to receive it.

"It's amazingly easy to shut someone else down," I said. "Without thinking about it we let pass countless occasions during the day when love makes a tentative appearance—in other words, we turn our backs on spirit. Your beloved may start to say something nice or give you an affectionate touch or ask how you are feeling. Notice how often this seed isn't allowed to grow, how quickly you simply cut the gesture off or take it for granted. In this way you limit the love you are receiving, rather than nurturing its faint beginnings."

"But I want Alan to love me," Jeanne said. "Why would I cut off the very thing I want?"

"Because negativity inside says no when love is offered. Look at your body language as well as your words, for you don't have to say the word *no* to shut Alan down. Do you detect a tendency to shrug, contract, bow your head, or turn away when he tries to be loving? Keep the following thought in mind for similar situations:

> *Being shown a gesture of love is like being offered a portion of God.*

"Look into the eyes of your beloved and learn to believe that love is really there. The ego, with all its fears and self-interests, blocks your ability to perceive the portion of God that your beloved is offering you. Eventually your expectations become self-fulfilling; the more you shut down gestures of love, the less motivated your beloved will be to make them.

"It isn't easy to stop sending these automatic turnoff signals, but you can take the first step by refusing to believe that *no* when someone else sees you as lovable. Once you stop shutting love down, it will become easier to let *no* be replaced by *yes*. This change shouldn't be forced. Allow Alan to pay attention to you as much as he wants, without manipulation or rejection. Start talking more about love in general with all those who are loving toward you—they will enjoy this topic more than you realize."

We were near the end of our time together, but Jeanne was a different person from the woman who had walked in—she had the look of someone much happier with herself. In parting I said, "When you find a genuinely loving person, as you have, you will see that you are in his heart not because you look a certain way or act a certain way, but because he is following his own nature—loving others is just the easiest way he knows how to be. When you realize this, the whole problem of not deserving is exposed for the illusion it really is."

# INFATUATION

When attraction reaches its peak, the phase known as infatuation begins. It is the most delirious stage of love—immortalized by Romeo and Juliet, Cyrano de Bergerac, and a thousand screen lovers —but it is also the most controversial. It is a time of extravagant emotions and wild optimism. Awareness of boundaries and limitations collapses, replaced by impossible idealism, at least as seen by an outside observer. To her family Juliet was not the sun or the moon, and Romeo's obsession with her was a danger to a young girl's virtue and safety.

But outside standards matter not at all in this phase. Infatuated lovers dwell so single-mindedly on their intoxicated emotions that they can hardly eat or sleep, their work becomes only a distraction from their consuming love.

Infatuation may be so extreme because it is a release from the loveless constriction we call normal. In spiritual terms, being infatuated means seeing another person as God, a divine being to be worshiped. In ancient India, to truly see the divine and be bathed in its radiance was called *Bhakti,* or devotion. From the devotional hymns of the Rig Veda, the oldest record of human worship, to the present, bhakti has been far and away the most popular means of approaching God. Religious worship, in the form of prayers, offerings, and celebrations, is an all-consuming affair for a true bhakta, who asks nothing more than to be intoxicated by the Lord.

In the Old Testament, when the poet of the Song of Solomon rhapsodizes about his love for God, his words gush as romantically as if he were swooning over a woman:

> You split me, tore my heart
>   open, filled me with love.
> You poured your spirit into me;
>   I knew you as I know myself.

The parallel between a lover's intoxication and a saint's is impossible to miss. It is in this phase of infatuation that lovers say they worship each other. "I am in love with loving," St. Augustine declares, echoing the passions of a million secular lovers.

What makes romantic love seem so religious is this sense of merging. The pouring of one spirit into another produces a ravishing ecstasy at its most intense. Perhaps no word is more recurrent during the delirium of infatuation than *new*. The release from old boundaries is like a birth that makes all things new.

The source of this newness is not a new person, however, but a shift in perception. The sensation of merging with another person comes about in the brain. To date we have no biochemical explanation for the suddenness and strength of this shift, although researchers have found that neuropeptides associated with intense pleasure, in particular serotonin, are elevated in lovers. Enhanced immune response in lovers is also well known to medical researchers. Yet the scientific paradigm is hardly able to account for the way romantic love can abolish the walls of separation that define the self. There is an irreversible trend from early infancy to create a stronger and stronger distinction between entities called "me" and "you." Normally we don't think of the natural separation between "me" and "you" as a source of suffering. Yet no agony is worse for the bhakta, or devotee, than to be away from God. In romance too the release from separation is so liberating that it has the power of a religious illumination.

This is not to say that everyone who falls in love falls this hard.

Sometimes attraction builds slowly, and other times the infatuation may be one-sided. When the object of love doesn't respond, infatuation becomes a self-centered preoccupation with fantasy. Spiritual masters have declared, however, that even when love is returned one is truly inspired by one's own higher Self. The reason that the word *Self* is more appropriate than the word *soul* is that it accentuates how love's journey is totally contained within one's own being.

The insights of this phase center on the ecstatic merging of self and Self:

> *Merging with another person is illusion; merging with the Self is supreme reality.*

> *If infatuation is madness, sanity pales beside it.*

> *The infatuated vision of lovers is like the holy vision of saints.*

## BETWEEN TWO WORLDS

Curiously, falling in love has a poor reputation among psychologists, going back to Freud, who fiercely ridiculed the spiritual meaning of romance. He viewed it as a primitive regression—his term for any retreat from adult self-control to infantile instincts and drives. Regression had previously been exalted as sacred, at least in literary circles. The greatest of English Romantic poets, William Wordsworth, articulated a common belief that childhood is the holiest time of life. Wordsworth describes a divinely inspired condition of infancy, when we are still bathed in light from the celestial world before birth:

> And not in utter nakedness,
> But trailing clouds of glory do we come
> From God, who is our home.

By being born, Wordsworth believed, an infant drops into a darker world, but for a while the perception of holiness lingers; as he goes on to say, "Heaven lies about us in our infancy," meaning that the state of innocence itself turns earth into a paradise. By some fortunate chance Wordsworth himself could still recall that earliest time when his surroundings were "apparelled in celestial light." But the loss of this radiant innocence had to come, as it does for all: "At length the Man perceives it die away,/and fade into the light of common day."

The condition described here pertains equally as well to newborn love. Ordinarily, a form of spiritual amnesia blots out the knowledge that we were ever in the light; this forgetfulness parallels the growth of a tough skin called ego that screens out knowledge that cannot be verified by the five senses. Until, that is, the second birth of innocence, called infatuation. Like a newborn child, the infatuated lover sees through eyes that make the world holy.

Modern child psychology supports this notion. As far as neurophysiologists can tell, infants do feel awash in a sea of oneness. Without boundaries or ego restraints, they are little gods in their worlds, their every need met simply by crying and reaching out, their self-centeredness so complete that every other person and thing is a mere extension of an all-pervading awareness of themselves.

Feeling totally merged with your environment would seem to serve no evolutionary purpose for a species, since it eliminates the possibility of defending yourself. Recently it was discovered, however, that humans are born with much more complete brains than we possess in adulthood. The threadlike connections, called dendrites, that branch off from every neuron are far more numerous just after birth than in any later stage of life. Dendrites are filaments of communication between brain cells, and presumably their oversupply at birth contributes to a baby's sense of being enveloped in a sea of sights, sounds, tastes, textures, and smells. From billions of bits of sensory data, the infant begins to select, to discriminate. As the range of reality gets narrowed down, like a radio band instead of one wash of noise, multitudes of dendrites are no longer needed.

In short, we pare down reality until we can handle it in rational terms, as neat slices of sensory data. Wordsworth was probably entirely accurate when he remembered a world bathed in light, for a baby's eyes could very likely see that way.

But this does not explain why lovers—and saints—revert to such a "primitive" perception. What makes infatuation so dubious to a rationalist—many psychologists won't even grant it the dignity of being called love—is that lovers return to a state devoid of useful discriminations. But from the spiritual perspective what seems like a primitive regression may be a *primal* one instead. Love's gift is to strip away a lifetime of imprints in the psyche that condition us to believe in separateness, returning us to the reality we were born in, which contains only love.

All of us have been conditioned since childhood to believe in a material world that can be verified by the senses. Lovers, being no different from the rest of us in this regard, often report that they live in two worlds, swept away by an overwhelming sense of merging and at the same time rationalizing that it can't be real. The beloved isn't an enchanted being; the world is not bathed in perfection's light—this must all be temporary insanity. Now comes the most delicate moment of all, for two opposed perceptions are warring within, and only one will survive.

The problem is that both are true. How can two perceptions of the same event be equally valid? This is one of the key issues in any spiritual event, because *perception is a choice.* The psychological description of falling in love is so opposed to the spiritual that they hardly seem to fit the same phenomenon.

Falling in love is

| Psychological | Spiritual |
|---|---|
| Temporary | Timeless |
| Illusory | Transcendent |
| Excited | Peaceful |
| Attached | Freeing |
| Hormone-based | Soul-based |
| Imaginary unity | Real unity |
| Childish regression | Enhanced evolution |

You do not have to go much further than this list to understand why even the most timeless of experiences, one that exposes the soul and opens the heart to bliss, doesn't survive very long. Arrayed against it is an entire worldview in which such things are not acknowledged as real. Not only are most people unprepared for the opening of spirit but they have been actively conditioned against it by the materialism that gave rise to modern psychology, stripping love of any "higher" meaning.

Love, however, has the power to unite our two worlds. Metaphysics says that the world is both immanent and transcendent. *Immanent* means "material, changing, subject to time." *Transcendent* means "eternal, timeless, and beyond the material." The lover sees a more real world because he or she looks at ordinary things and finds the spiritual light that is actually there. The rest of us miss the transcendent and therefore claim it doesn't exist; we are doing the best we can, yet we cannot claim truth for our side.

The mystery is not whether you will begin to transcend your old reality when you fall in love, for that is certain. What is mysterious is that being engulfed in your beloved is also divine. But the visitation of spirit is a subtle phenomenon, and a very impatient one. Either spirit takes you with it or it quickly departs.

Transcendence comes in many forms. Astronauts awed by the sight of the earth, a blue pearl hovering against the blackness of the universe, have transcended; the first mountaineers to scale the Alps recorded the transcendent exaltation of their experience. In other words, falling in love is not as unique as it may feel; in fact it is the most common of transcending experiences, given how few of us go up in space or ascend the Matterhorn. Common insights link all these peak experiences: one feels that life is a blessed state, that fear is unreal because death is not an extinction but merely a transition, that love surrounds and nourishes us all, and that some part of ourselves lives beyond the world of struggle and care, in the domain of pure existence.

From a spiritual point of view, infatuation opens us up to these same insights—the beloved serves as a trigger, like the mountain, the space walk, the near-death encounter. This is not to diminish the allure of the beloved, for the transcendent wonder of infatuation has no difficulty shining through the physical delight—in love, the immanent and the transcendent are one.

# LOVING PRACTICE

## Seeing Beyond

Not only infatuated lovers have a sense of living in two worlds. The literal meaning of *transcending* is "going beyond," and at moments of clarity it is possible for anyone to be aware that reality isn't confined to the five senses. Peak experiences open up windows to spirit. Yet "going beyond" is not an accurate description of the experience of transcending, since there is no distance to cover; spirit never leaves us, it is only overlooked.

This practice trains you to stop overlooking the spirit and love that surround you, waiting to be noticed.

Although it means "going beyond," a better way to describe transcending is "seeing beyond." What can you see beyond the apparently solid facade of life, the constant flow of time, the limitations of space, and the laws of cause and effect? If the answer is very little, the reason is that your perception has not been trained for such vision. Yet every day contains clues of the second reality we all inhabit, which is timeless, unbounded, causeless, and intimately tied to our needs on the path to love.

First examine the following list to determine if you have experienced these sorts of clues:

1. In the midst of danger or crisis, have you suddenly had the feeling of being completely safe and protected?
2. Have you been with someone who was dying and felt a sense of peace or a coolness in the air when the moment of passing came?
3. Have you known someone who recovered from an "incurable" illness?
4. Have you prayed and had your prayer answered?
5. Have you ever witnessed a soft light around another person or yourself?
6. Have you ever asked for silent guidance or the answer to a dilemma and received it?
7. When looking at a sunset, a full moon, or something of great natural beauty, have you felt yourself expand as if you were no longer enclosed within the physical limits of your body?
8. Have you experienced a silencing of your mind, perhaps just before going to sleep or on first waking up?
9. Have you felt a loving presence when you most needed it?
10. Do you ever hear an inner voice you feel you can absolutely rely on? (This voice doesn't have to speak in words; it can also be a strong feeling or intuition.)
11. Have you felt wonder at the sight of a newborn child?

This isn't a quiz. You aren't trying to answer yes to as many questions as possible, but if you did say yes to any of them, pick the one that resonated most for you. Let us say it was the first one: feeling a sudden sense of safety and protection in the midst of crisis or danger. Close your eyes and put yourself back into that situation; see all the details of where you were, who you were with, what time it was, and so on. Try to relive the moment, but instead of being the person who was reacting at that moment, ask to be given a larger perspective. Ask to see the meaning of what was happening, and request that the meaning be as specific as possible. Take a deep breath and listen to whatever response comes.

If you do not get a specific answer, ask for all blocks to the truth to be removed, and take another deep breath. Does an image come to mind, a story, a phrase? Whatever comes, take it to be your answer. If you get only confusion or resistance, relax and wait a moment.

Now interpret your answer. Do any of the following meanings come through?

> I am loved.
> I am safe.
> A part of my self watches over me.
> I know.
> I am.
> The light is with me.
> God is real. God is.
> Nothing is wrong.
> I am at peace.
> Things are OK.
> I can love.
> Everything is one.

These are the messages that love is trying to send you at every moment. Each is extremely simple yet eternally true. You do not have to have an extraordinary or peak experience to receive such messages, but peak experiences do bring sudden clarity. The walls of old conditioning, habits, and expectations drop away at such moments.

None of these messages has to come through literally as described above. Perhaps at the bedside of a dying person you felt a warm glow in your heart and a sense of calmness. This can be interpreted in many ways—pick the one that fits your experience most closely.

Go through your most vivid experiences of spirit, soul, God, or love, and again look for messages that they may have contained for you. Having done this with your memories, you are now ready to apply the same technique to the present.

*Attune yourself to spirit, and it will speak to you in love.*

Spirit isn't a phenomenon; it is the whispered truth within a phenomenon. As such, spirit is gentle, it persuades by the softest touch. The messages never get louder, only clearer. If you have the slightest hint of communication from spirit, ask for clarification; look at the preceding list if you need to. At first the links to spirit may seem tenuous and fragile, but as you grow more confident, you will find that your life is full of meaning, that every moment has an aspect that goes beyond if you have the vision to find it.

# In Our Lives

## ... But Never the Bride

Clare is one of the few people you'll meet who has never complained about her love life. The truth is that she is rarely *not* in love. As a teenager she covered the walls of her bedroom with glossy photos of Hollywood leading men, falling in love with each in turn. After she grew up she continued to be easily smitten, and her attitude toward any man she had fallen for—warm, admiring, a bit timid, yet eager to find out all about him—won her a great deal of attention in return.

But Clare was also ruthless. She would tear down the photos of any heartthrob who slipped from her high expectations, and this is true of her today. A man has to be powerful, well off, handsome, and self-assured even to attract her notice. Few have been able to live up to her ideal of a "perfect" lover. In college Clare had a few discreet affairs with her professors, preferring older men who had achieved academic recognition. This was not difficult to do, since she was attending a prestigious Boston women's college, but afterward she continued to gravitate toward married men. Within a few years Clare found that not many women approached her with anything but feelings of distrust and suspicion.

She barely noticed. While circulating as a young journalist among the politicians and power brokers of Boston, she was in a perpetual glow of infatuation. Clare had a knack for bringing out the best in any man she was smitten by—which made her a top-notch interviewer. Her subtle surrenders brought the charm out in men who actually possessed very little.

The only flaw in her love life was that it wasn't real—few of these powerful men ever came home with her, and no relationship extended beyond a few months of hit-and-run hotel stays. Ten years passed. All of her friends from college had gotten married. Clare continued to live in fantasies that faded once her "perfect" men turned out to be fallible after all.

"Is it my fault if they all let me down?" she mourned. Increasingly she became aware of a lingering sense of loneliness; after getting burned by an older man in public office whose wife detected their affair, Clare sought fewer opportunities for seduction, except in fantasy.

Fantasy can be exciting and diverting, but it is almost never associated with insight. In fact, Clare seems to use her fantasies of a perfect lover to preclude any possibility that she might see into herself. Her obstacle in life appeared to be that the right men were all unavailable, but in truth she picked them *because* they were un-available. Ensuring in advance that there is a fatal flaw in your partner makes it easy to reject before you get rejected yourself. In this regard Clare was a master.

When I met with Clare, as part of a teaching workshop on healing, she was full of opinions about how men have lower spiritual vibrations, about how uncomfortable she is in the presence of lower-chakra energies, and the like. "Then why do you fall for so many men in the first place?" I asked. She looked taken aback.

"I don't think this is so much about what's going on with men as it is with you," I said. Clare has a genuine commitment to her healing work, and I felt we could talk frankly about her fears and inner wounds. I suggested that we explore the issue of fear and fantasy, since the two are so closely intertwined.

"In your situation fear of commitment seems to be critical, especially since your chief complaint is that men don't commit to you," I said.

"I can't be responsible for that," Clare protested. "They come and they go. It's their choice."

"But this is a reflection of a fear you may not be facing in yourself. Fear of commitment comes in many forms. But what does it say spiritually?"

*Fear of commitment mirrors a belief that spirit is unreachable.*
*Thus, love becomes hopeless.*

Clare's situation speaks of underlying isolation and despair. From her I got the impression of a woman in a double bind, constantly asking for love but making sure that those she asked were not in a position to respond on any but the most superficial level. It didn't surprise me that Clare's father was extremely unavailable. Born into a working-class family in San Francisco, he had risen from being a dockhand on the Embarcadero wharves to being president of his own shipping company. He had become a hero to four generations of his family, from his Italian immigrant grandparents to his own children. But the qualities that made him "great"—his power, drive, magnetism, and shrewdness—also made him very forbidding. None of these qualities is lovable, yet they were all Clare had when she was growing up. Her solution was to *make* them lovable.

The first person she had a crush on was her father, and in essence she has repeated that romance over and over, finding men to "love" for their success and status when in fact she has been mortally afraid of approaching anyone who has real love to offer.

"When a powerful man takes notice of you," I asked, "how do you feel?"

"Special. Cared for. Important," Clare shot back without hesitation.

"But isn't this importance and specialness coming by proxy?" I asked. "What you need is to have your 'ordinariness' deemed special." Clare looked confused. I asked her to write down this sentence: *Spirit loves me for simply being here.* "If you can begin to believe this one thing," I said, "the man you attract as a lover will hold the same attitude."

Ironically, Clare is a glutton for love if it comes with the charge of power, but moments of quiet, gentleness, solitude, intimate rapport, and murmured endearments secretly bore her, leaving her feeling that something is missing. Spiritually these are the moments when each of us has a chance to find love in all its splendid simplicity; but for Clare the emptiness she feels whenever things quiet down allows the grief of an abandoned child to rise too near the surface.

Reading Clare's story in symbolic spiritual terms is very helpful. In her father we see a powerful, remote God who demands to be worshiped. This image has been easily transposed onto the men in Clare's life. It's not hard to see that she is in a spiritual predicament, mirrored on all sides by the situations she keeps creating.

The fact that Clare seizes on every opportunity to fall in love tells me that she craves a spiritual opening; only when madly infatuated does she feel wanted in this world, cared for by a higher power. Everything else is a disappointment. The problem is that the opening to spirit keeps closing, since Clare actually resents and fears higher power. How can she replace her old, unsuccessful pattern?

"You're here this weekend to talk about healing," I said, "and in your case, physical and emotional healing would be superficial. Your need is for a healing at the level of belief."

"Meaning what?" she asked.

"I suppose we could say you need a better love life with God. First your concept of 'higher' power has to be reexamined. God or spirit stands beside us in every aspect of our everyday lives. Second, the belief that God is masculine must be exchanged for a genderless alternative, given how threatening masculine energy is to you. If you can begin to see how your notion of spirit has been shaped by your early childhood, you can start to look at love as a mirror of the present instead of the past." This last is a key concept:

> *When you fall in love, you fall for a mirror of your own most present needs.*

The intense desirability of another person isn't innate in that person. Desire is born in the one who desires. In Clare's case, since her underlying self-image is that of a helpless, unloved girl, any show of power arouses incredible yearning in her.

There is nothing wrong with this—we all project similar needs in our search for love. Nor is there anything wrong with the bedazzled state of infatuation that Clare has so often sought. Each affair, real or imaginary, has a repeated message to offer her: "You are loved." It is the simplest of messages, but often the hardest to absorb. For spirit isn't saying, "You are loved as long as your passion for this man lasts." It is saying, "You are loved," without any qualifications. If Clare does begin to gain insight and remove the obstacles that block her vision, spirit's message will be awaiting her. There is infinite patience in spirit, infinite willingness to wait upon our attention. And one day, in her own time, Clare will notice.

"I think that each man you have loved is a tiny reminder of who you are," I told Clare. "This isn't solipsistic but a natural reflection of your needs. You aren't judged by the love life you choose, since no one is outside yourself to judge—there is only you as the Self, looking at you from a different angle."

"I don't see how that helps," Clare said.

"The Self looking at you is the primary relationship you bring into all situations," I said. "Realizing that, you will start to reduce expectations for other relationships. In your case you expect a lot from fantasy, but you could transfer those expectations to yourself. What do you really want from men? Security, well-being, a sense of belonging? These are all available to you from your own Self, and your healing will be to fall in love with that Self."

The secret to spiritual healing is that its foundation is already laid. In his exalted poetry, Walt Whitman speaks of the ever-presentness of love:

> There was never any more inception than there is now,
> Nor any more youth or age than there is now,
> And will never be any more perfection than there is now,
> Nor any more heaven or hell than there is now.

I read this passage to Clare, who sat silently for a moment. "I've been around for a while," she said, "and I'm not unconscious. I see that I'm stuck, and for a long time this concept of learning to love yourself has been prescribed to me. But I honestly cannot see how it works."

"The reason for that," I said, "is that you are bringing the wrong model to your notion of what self-love is. In duality, love connects two separate people. If that is your model of love, you will have no choice but to see self-love in much the same way. That is, you'll try to separate off the parts of yourself that you value and direct appreciation toward them. But fragmentation is the problem, not the solution. Self-love and self-division don't go together. Self-love isn't on the level of personality; it's on the level of being. Being is whole, and when you recognize that, every part of yourself rejoins its true status as totality. Learning to love and accept the powerless, lonely little girl inside you, giving her permission to be part of you, will lessen her role in directing your love life."

If you strip away the details of Clare's story, her search for love in all the wrong places stands for a much more general condition. Love between "you" and "me" is a dualistic conception. People have been falling madly in love for centuries, but that hasn't solved the deeper problem of inner division. If anything, such division has been exacerbated as generation after generation tries to resolve separation through others. What heals inner division is a change of perception.

You are not just a small piece of divine essence that was created to exist separately. At the level of your soul you are the whole of spirit. Your connection to God is complete and seamless; your loving relationship to the universe is total. The mind cannot conceive of this all-inclusiveness, however, while being caught in its own dualism. We think of ourselves as father *or* mother, son *or* daughter, man *or* woman, here *or* there, this *or* that. Separation is built from our own self-image.

Thought cannot restore wholeness because by definition thought is also fragmented. Yet everyone's mind contains the essence of spirit; silence and intuitive knowledge come naturally to us. The fact that we have drastically devalued these aspects of our inner life doesn't abolish them. Already you can touch on valuable parts of your life that you can know only by setting thoughts aside. How do you know if you are happy, or intelligent, or awake? These aren't issues you reason with; they are self-evident.

You do not have to think in order to see and hear; you do not have to have an active dialogue inside your head to know that you exist.

*Awareness is aware of itself before it gains knowledge of anything else.*

The deeper reaches of intuitive knowledge, however, feel foreign because our culture hasn't shown us how to explore the inner world. When we turn to privileged outsiders—to seers and poets, for example—we discover many truths that only the silent voice of spirit can reveal. If we could rise above our narrowness of vision, we would perceive our higher Self directly, as Walt Whitman did:

> There is that in me—I do not know what it is—but I
> know it is in me. . . .
> Do you see O my brothers and sisters?
> It is not chaos or death—it is form, union, plan—it is
> eternal life—it is Happiness.

The fact that we cannot sustain Whitman's vision means that our growth from duality to unity is still under way, which is why the path to love exists. The ability to live in the Self must be relearned—this is what walking the path is all about.

# TENDER COURTSHIP

The next stage of romance, courtship, is more than just the time for winning one's love. At a subtler level it brings together two people's perceptions. Beneath the lovers' talk and tender emotions, the fragile birth of spirit is being tested. Its survival depends not just on how exalted and transformed a man and woman may feel. An act of interpretation must also take place, in which the right words are found for a shared experience.

Courtship is a tender, tentative stage in which two lovers decide whether to pursue a new reality or return to the old. It is the first phase in which two futures are at stake, not just one.

In ancient India the spiritual equivalent of this phase was called *Satsang,* a word that can be translated as "the company of truth," or more loosely, "the sharing of spirit." When disciples sat at the feet of their master, listening to his wisdom, they were taking satsang, but any communion of spiritual seekers is given the same name. Before departing this world, Christ told his disciples, "Where two or three of you gather in my name, I will be there." That is satsang without the master's physical presence. Turning your conversation in the direction of spirit makes a casual chat with a friend a form of satsang as well. The link with courtship is very clear, for courtship is about speaking your heart to another, sharing your spirit in a way you cannot do alone.

The satsang of lovers often takes place in silence, which holds true for some of the greatest saints also; simply to be in their presence infuses us with the spirit of God. People who feel genuinely comfortable with each other are able to talk about their fears, wishes, and hopes, but the communion of lovers is far more intense. Courtship is a shared birth, a rare opportunity to exchange what is most innocent in each partner. Intimacy allows a man to tell a woman things he did not know existed within himself, and the same for a woman.

What becomes shared may have never existed in the past. The past is based on memory, which will always remain personal. Up to the point when they merged, two lovers walked separate paths. Together they create a new path that has no past, where every step moves into the unknown, and no amount of experience can light the way.

The following are the insights brought about in love's first communion:

> *Awareness can be shared. What God gives you out of love, you can give to someone you love.*

> *Communion is the basis of trust.*

> *The unknown is the territory of lovers.*

## A STRUGGLE BETWEEN LOVE AND EGO

When two people meet in satsang, they can bring the fullness of their higher Selves, yet what most of us bring to courtship is not fullness but need. When need dominates over love the fragile thread of spirit is broken. Need implies a lack in oneself, a missing piece that someone else must supply. Women are generally asked to supply the softness, nurturing, comfort, beauty, and affection that men cannot otherwise find within. Men are expected to supply the strength, protection, power, and will that women cannot otherwise find. Both feel that the other has made them complete.

Need is a powerful thing, capable of creating powerful illusions.

No one can really enter you and replace a missing piece. The softness or tenderness or nurturing a man finds in a woman is only borrowed unless he can be taught to develop those same qualities. A woman may benefit from the power, will, and strength she finds in a man, but that is not the same as having these qualities become her own.

In courtship we decide whether to borrow from another or actually become what the other represents. In communion you can become what you perceive, if your satsang is deep enough. It is all a question of intent. Will you bandage your inner needs or actually heal them? Only the long journey ahead can answer this, but courtship clears the way.

Given our cultural conditioning, most couples lose the fragile thread of spirit in this phase. As the heightened emotions of infatuation begin to cool, what replaces them is ego, the main component of the false self. We all rely upon our egos to lead us through the known world. "I" is not a fixed entity but a constantly accumulating set of experiences.

The ego always seems to know what it needs. An ego need can be defined as anything that bolsters "me." By feeding your isolated identity, you continue the most familiar mode of existence you have known, which is the pursuit of self-image. The fact that romantic passion can take a person beyond ego doesn't abolish the ego's needs.

Typically, the courtship phase is when most lovers begin to have doubts. The issue of commitment arises, and the first hints of incompatibility make their unwelcome appearance. Courtships generally break off when one or the other person feels that his or her needs aren't going to be met. The man may feel that the woman is not sufficiently deferential or supportive of his self-image; the woman may feel that the man is not sensitive or caring enough to nourish her feelings.

Although it is typical for both a man and a woman to have potent fantasies about each other before they become intimate, once they begin to spend time together, fantasy is not strong enough to restrain the ego. There is now a precarious balance between love, which makes communion possible, and need, which doesn't want to sacrifice selfishness unless forced to.

It is unfair to blame any single person for lack of trust given our social experience. We have all been conditioned to obey ego needs blindly. We are a society that has grown suspicious of intimate contact. Some intrusions of personal space are horrifying, such as rape and murder, but the betrayal of space is extremely disturbing even when violence isn't done. Two people engaged in an alimony fight or a bitter custody dispute are in essence taking advantage of the intimate knowledge they gained in marriage, turning trust into aggression. It is no wonder that allowing another person past your well-guarded defenses causes deep conflict, for the person who might deliver you from threat might also prove to be the enemy inside your gates.

Being in love isn't going to abolish crime, war, homelessness, racial strife, and the multitude of other threats around us. The ego uses these outside dangers to convince you that the world is hostile and uncaring. To all appearances the ego is right, but only according to its isolationist perspective. In truth, to see anything without love is to see it fearfully. Threat doesn't arise "out there." Its origins are "in here," where we first establish our beliefs. Defenses exist to ward off threat. They are like an early warning system that can be tuned so sensitively that *no one* could be unthreatening enough to disarm them.

The real question, then, is how to defuse the sense of threat enough to allow love to be trusted. What feeds threat and keeps it going? The answers are many, but they can be simplified. Every threat is a shadow from the past.

*In reality there is nothing to fear in the present. Fear is
projected onto the present by memory.*

Newborn infants, because they have no past, lack all defenses; a
baby is completely vulnerable to any intruder or harmful influence,
utterly dependent upon outside protection to survive. Yet, paradoxi-
cally, no one is more invulnerable than a newborn child, because it
has no fear. Experience has yet to create its imprint on the nervous
system, and without a frame of reference there is no threat. (It is true
that babies have instinctive fears, such as fear of falling, but these are
physical rather than psychological. Physical fear contributes to survival, whereas psychological fear can be crippling. The one promotes
fast, sure reactions; the other can create paralysis.)

Threat is a subjective interpretation that must be taught; it often
bears little relationship to the actual danger surrounding a person.
That is why a sport like mountain climbing can turn instinctive fear—
the fear of falling—into a joyful experience; everything depends
upon interpretation.

The enterprise of learning how to defend oneself in the world
takes a long time. We all cherish our survival skills, having long ago
abandoned the fearlessness of a newborn. When courtship asks us to
commit ourselves to another person, we unconsciously see this as a
decision that could affect our survival—that is what giving up your
defenses feels like. Your doubt and mistrust toward someone you
love is a mirror of your own belief that fear is necessary, that survival
isn't possible without defenses.

## SEPARATING TRUE FROM FALSE

Courtship allows trust to grow despite old wounds. Given how many
years we've all spent building our defenses, this healing doesn't hap-

pen quickly. In fact, the first phase of healing brings up old wounds to be felt afresh. Only when you begin to feel safe does your psyche permit you to look at fears that were too intense to confront before. It is common for either partner to relive, in contemporary form, the traumas and survival threats of childhood. It isn't surprising, then, that a man and woman may not permit themselves to be in a healing relationship at first. They need the courage to see that the doubt and fear that surface at odd moments is coming up to be examined and released, not blindly acted on.

The most destructive effect of feeling threatened is to cut off the flow of love. If you were not taught about love from childhood, being able to be undefended with another person is much more difficult. Loving parents must teach their children that reality isn't simply harsh.

*All of us were imprinted one of two ways: either the world is dangerous with moments of safety, or the world is safe with moments of danger.*

No matter how hostile the world appears, a loving family remains secure as a place of nurturing and protection. Children don't need to trust everyone, only someone who will never let them down— thus the original balance between love and need is established. A strong positive imprint from infancy can last a lifetime. Even though only two parents taught a child to love, it is as if the whole world loved that child, and the belief "I am loved" endures as part of his or her reality. When you have a rock-bottom belief that you are loved, your needs won't be so desperate; there will be room to allow another person into your inner space.

The worst imprint you can have from childhood is that your models for love were also models of betrayal. This happens in cases of abuse—physical, sexual, or emotional. With any sort of abuse in your background, you will secretly regard every lover as an enemy. The gentlest caress contains the possibility of being struck; the softest endearment resonates with potential degradation.

Ironically, it is just these children who grow up to crave love the most, but being insecure, feeling the need for defense beyond what is reasonable, they also pull away from commitment the fastest. Such people are not certain deep down that they can feel love, despite their craving for it. Even the most intoxicating romance will not be able to overcome a history that places ego needs much higher than those of relationship.

Getting to true love is a growth process, and the first requirement is to become aware of when you are not being true. Courtship provides an opportunity for creating this awareness, since this is when a couple work out their own definition of what being in love means. Many things pass for love that are something else. These forms of false love can be behaviors, beliefs, expectations, or conditioning from the past. We all tend to accept versions of "love" that we are used to, without stopping to examine their validity. Much unloving behavior gets past us in this way.

Perhaps no sentence in the English language contains as many hidden meanings as "I love you." Very often we say these words and silently add expectations that underline them. What we really are saying may be

> I love you as long as you stay the way you are now.
> I love you if you love me.
> I love you if you don't scare me too much.
> I love you as long as you do what I want.

Because these sentences all carry expectations, they are not really about love. "I love you" is often not a simple declaration but with unspoken conditions—"I love you if." People who make conditional promises are not wrong, they are usually doing the best they can. No doubt someone in their past said, "I love you," when what they really meant was "I love you if." To a greater or lesser degree we all place expectations upon the people we love. But these expectations, however reasonable they may seem to us, inject an element of false-ness that true love doesn't contain.

False love can also take the form of lack of realism. Someone who expects to be swept away by a mysterious stranger and rescued from all problems is indulging in unreality. Unreality has many disguises, of which fantasy and projection are the two most prevalent. Fantasy creates a false image that love is expected to live up to. We fantasize about an ideal lover, and anyone who does not match this ideal becomes unfit for our love. Being too old or too young, too tall or too short, too dull, too poor, too unprofessional—too anything that does not pass the test—this is how other people come to be seen as lacking potential for love. The root of this unreality clearly lies in the perceiver, however, not the perceived. The fantasy that supposedly pictures our ideal in fact puts on blinders.

Projection distorts our perception in a different way: it attaches our beliefs to other people. Someone who believes that no one will ever love him is projecting his own lack of acceptance onto others. The internal belief "I'm not lovable" is so painful that it cannot be faced, and one way to lessen that pain is to stop claiming it as your own. Instead you decide that other people are at fault. *They* have let you down, *they* don't think you are good enough, *they* have no wish to love you. In reality there is no *they*, only projection.

False love can take more forms than active fantasy or projection. It may simply be expressed as something missing in one's experience. If you have not been shown loving behavior, you will have no positive images to fill the heart. The cruelest impression that can be made on a young child is indifference, and it may be the most common. To ignore a child's need for love conveys to the heart that its need is not essential. Upon growing up such a child will find it very difficult to express real love. In place of a warm outflow of feeling, he or she will feel a cooler, more moderated emotion that too easily flickers and fails. Indifference has a long legacy.

All these versions of false love are extremely common. We exhibit false love whenever we pretend to love someone beyond what we actually feel, whenever we fail to trust or be honest, whenever we push away someone else's offered emotions. Like the thousand-headed serpent, false love has too many heads to name. Defeating it requires that we discover what true love is. It takes the real to drive out the unreal. Recognizing a fantasy or projection puts distance between you and it; once you have obtained some distance, you can begin to renounce the power of the false.

If in the past you haven't experienced love's purity and understood its innocence, then the foundation of relationship hasn't been laid. Longfellow spoke truly when he said, "Love gives itself; it isn't bought." If a man or woman feels there is a price to pay for being loved, their whole sense of love is damaged. It has become confused with a transaction between winners and losers in a game of competing needs.

Our society makes the problem worse by claiming that selfishness is justified, for the easiest disguise for fear and doubt is selfishness. What good do "higher" values really bring the "me" who has a hard enough time surviving as it is? A cynic might say, "When people fall in love, they indulge in an escapist fantasy. There is a much more powerful force than love, called desire. Desire comes down to the pursuit of sex, money, power, security, and comfort. These are what people *really want*."

On the surface the cynic appears to be absolutely right. Life doesn't lie, which means that although all of us may espouse love, we don't live it. Selfishness has too strong a claim. Too often courtship serves to lay the groundwork for mutual selfishness. A man and woman bypass the pain of exposing their deepest fears and insecurity. Instead of pursuing the delicate work of weaving the threads of love into a fabric that will be strong enough to hold, they concentrate on what the relationship will do for "me."

> *The courtship phase succeeds to the extent that a man and woman can dismantle their defenses; it fails to the extent that they build new defenses together.*

How many couples bond together by forming a "we" that is just a stronger, tougher version of "me"? We can't be surprised when this happens. If survival is paramount in a dangerous world, two are better at it than one. Like an individual, a couple can pursue power and money, or at the very least security and comfort. Love gets left behind because it won't bring material rewards, at least not as clearly as unloving tactics will. Money and power require toughness, the willingness to fight for what you want. You are better off having a killer instinct, not a loving heart, if you pursue these things. Security and comfort also require looking out for number one. In this case one has become two; nothing else has changed.

Undoubtedly mutual ego needs have a place in every relationship. The real problem occurs when they obliterate the tender growth of love in its spiritual aspect. Long before we fall in love, we know more than enough about our needs. Acquiring an ally to fulfill them isn't the same as getting free from them. Only love can free us, because its truth is an antidote to fear. The cynical claim that what people really want is money, power, and security falls apart once we look deeper. The exhilaration of falling in love is an escape from ego, its sense of threat, and its selfishness. This escape is what we *really* want. Whatever rewards it brings, the ego cannot do two things: it cannot abolish fear, since ego is founded on fear; and it cannot create love, since ego by definition shuts out love.

The reason that ego and love are not compatible comes down to this: you cannot take your ego into the unknown, where love wants to lead. If you follow love, your life will become uncertain, and the ego craves certainty. You will have to surrender to another person, and the ego prizes its own will above anyone else's. Love will make your feelings ambiguous, and the ego wants to feel the certainty of right and wrong. Many other experiences that cannot be comprehended by ego apply to love—a lover is confused, spontaneous, vulnerable, exposed, detached, carefree, wondrous, and ever new.

Love's journey would be terrifying if we didn't have passion to give us courage—the blind courage of lovers, it is often called. It would be truer to call it the blind wisdom of lovers, because the ego's certainty is an illusion. Uncertainty is the basis of life.

# LOVING PRACTICE

## Unpeeling the Layers of Love

One of the most valuable things you can learn about yourself is what you mean by the words "I love you." The meaning you impart is complex because it contains *you*. Your past associations with love, your childhood imprints, your unspoken expectations and beliefs are all packaged in language. Thus "I love you" expands into

"I love you the way my father loved my mother before
they got divorced."
"I love you as long as you don't get too close."
"I love you more than Romeo loved Juliet, but please
don't ask me to die."
"I love you the way the high school football captain didn't
love me."

Words become more personal the more emotional they are. Since "I love you" is the most emotional phrase in our language, it includes many feelings that you might never openly refer to, particularly painful ones. The meanings that get overlooked in everyday speech can be brought to the surface through the technique of association, which is the basis of this practice.

## PART ONE

Sit down with a pencil and paper and record your answers to this question.

What's the first name that comes to mind when you think of each of the following words?

Saintly

Passionate

Kind

Adventurous

Beautiful

Courageous

Tender

Loyal

Handsome

Selfless

Strong

Funny

Genius

Innocent

Admirable

Talented

Generous

Adorable

Naturally no two people produce anything like the same list of answers, but there are definite profiles of how lists are formed. Out of eighteen possible choices

➤ *If more than eight of your responses were fictional,* you have a strong fantasy component to your definition of love. This also holds true if movie and TV stars figure prominently on your list. You probably see a "perfect" lover as unattainable but intensely desirable. You look for external beauty before intrinsic qualities. You probably do not see yourself as beautiful, fascinating, or very worthy of the attention of people you admire.

➤ *If more than eight of your responses were people you've never met,* you have a strong streak of idealism in your definition of love. You may be dependent on hero worship to give you strength; you unconsciously see a lover as a rescuer, provider, tower of strength, father figure, or authority.

➤ *If more than five of your responses are your father or mother,* you have not formed a strong sense of love on your own but look to childhood models.

➤ *If more than five of your responses are "me,"* you are not honestly answering the quiz, indicating fear or insecurity about being loved.

➤ *If more than five of your responses are the same name,* you are probably in love with that person.

➤ *If your spouse doesn't appear in your answers at least three times,* you haven't fully confronted your doubts about your relationship. Opening new lines of communication is in order.

## PART TWO

Association is a remarkably telling thing. In a classic experiment from the 1920s, a Russian filmmaker named Lev Kuleshov projected some simple images—a bowl of soup, a coffin, and a baby playing with a teddy bear—and after each image the blank face of a man looking at the camera. When this sequence was shown, audiences "read" all kinds of meaning into the man's expression. When it appeared after the bowl of soup, they thought he was hungry; after the coffin, he was afraid of dying; and after the baby, he felt love. These interpretations show just how powerful association can be.

The way your mind ties things together by association is often just as misleading. The fact is that we rarely see people for who they are; we see them by association with people from our past. For example, we carry around in our heads the physical images of our parents and match them to everyone we meet. Too close a resemblance provokes associations, good and bad, that have nothing to do with these new people and everything to do with our own mental processes.

I mentioned earlier that false love operates by projection, displacing your own feelings upon another. In the Kuleshov experiment, if a viewer of the film said that the man with the blank face hated the baby, projection was at work. But there is also a different kind of projection, based on your own desires. You might see someone as trustworthy, for example, because you need him to be that way (a reflection of having been betrayed in the formative past), and no matter how many times that person proves that he cannot be trusted, you will continue to project your need upon him. Jealousy involves extremes of projection and is difficult to dispel, since an innocent look or an innocent word can so easily be misinterpreted.

If you resort to projection a lot, you will tend to exhibit the following behavior:

> You finish people's sentences for them.
> You act defensive before being accused.
> You use verbal formulas such as "He's the kind of person who" and "I just know she's going to."
> You ask someone's opinion and then get angry if it disagrees with yours.
> You have a hard time reading other people's faces.
> You frequently feel misunderstood.
> You see threat in the faces of authority figures like

policemen, or feel that your boss secretly dislikes you, even though she has never said so.

You believe that when your spouse looks at another man (or woman), sexual interest is being shown.

You harbor extreme likes or dislikes for people you barely know.

Getting rid of projection is critical if you want to be able to tell true love from false, as either the giver or the receiver.

*Projection always hides a feeling you don't want to look at.*

If you examine any negative trait you insist is present in another person, you will find the same trait hiding in yourself. The more you deny this trait, the more strongly you will have to project it. Thus if you habitually defend yourself before being accused, you feel guilty. That guilt needs to be faced in order to stop the projection. If you feel that the man or woman you love is constantly looking at others with sexual interest, you are the one who cannot be trusted. If you think your boss secretly hates you, look at the possibility that you have hidden rage against authority. The following exercise is a good step toward honest self-evaluation.

Make a list of three people whom you intensely dislike, disapprove of, or have had strong conflicts with. Put down four qualities for each that you find most offensive. A typical list might look like this:

*Father-in-law:* arrogant, greedy, small-minded, bullheaded
*Boss:* unfair, temperamental, unappreciative of my work, inefficient
*Hitler:* sadistically cruel, hateful, prejudiced, fanatical

Now look at the list, and for each trait say, "I acted like that when I . . ." Finish the sentence with an example of your own behavior. When were you arrogant? When were you greedy? The point is not to wallow in self-criticism but to bring home feelings that need reclaiming instead of displacing them onto others.

If you have been honest with your list, you will find it very difficult to finish some sentences. Hitler's sadism, for example, may seem far removed from your behavior, or your boss's unfairness in not promoting you may be too fresh a wound. But by persevering you will discover that what you hate most in others you most strongly deny in yourself. This is a spiritual truth that we try to evade by projecting, blaming, and making excuses for ourselves. When you are able to see yourself in what you hate, you come closer to realizing that you contain everything, as befits a child of spirit.

# In Our Lives

## Cinderella for Sale

The first day that Dana came to work for Stephen, a spark passed between them. Fifteen years older than she and a highly successful plastic surgeon, Stephen didn't stand on ceremony. He told Dana that she didn't have to call him "Doctor" unless a patient was present, and when he asked about her background, he showed flattering interest. Dana had returned to technicians' school in her midtwenties. This was her first job since graduation, and the fact that Stephen offered her a generous pay package increased her eagerness to work for him.

Within a month he asked her for a date. Dana was nervous, afraid that the other women in the office would be antagonized, but Stephen put on a full-court press. After dinner at a fine French restaurant, he sent flowers the next morning. More dates followed, and although Dana found it difficult to warm up to an older man as a romantic partner, she had to agree with him that age is only in your head. Being around her seemed to make Stephen young again, as he was fond of telling Dana. But regardless of the good it did him, Stephen made sure that his wooing put Dana in the spotlight.

He sent flowers to her apartment nearly every day, and bought her expensive jewelry, which at first Dana was embarrassed to accept;

she gave in only because her refusal caused Stephen such obvious pain. In time they made the transition to sexual partners. Stephen was an attentive lover, although Dana got the impression he would be sensitive to any criticism or even suggestion about his performance. She therefore was more passive and compliant than she would have been with another man—it seemed a small sacrifice to make.

Stephen had grown children by his first marriage, which had taken place in medical school. Neither of them seemed eager to meet Dana, who was little more than ten years older than Stephen's son, a freshman in college. Stephen's divorce had been granted three years before, but Stephen had little to say about his first wife, even when asked for details. Nothing seemed to exist for him outside Dana, and she couldn't help but be immensely flattered.

They had met in June, and by early autumn a wedding date was set for Christmas. After buying Dana a huge engagement ring, Stephen urged her to buy the best of everything for the ceremony. They planned a lavish honeymoon in Paris—or rather, Stephen planned it and sprang the news on Dana. She was a little distressed by not having been consulted, but it was hard to utter the slightest complaint in the face of Stephen's overwhelming generosity.

The bubble didn't burst all at once. The first hint that something went wrong came when Stephen gave Dana an exercise video for tightening the muscles of her bottom—women were prone to softness there, he said, even when they looked as sensational as Dana. A week later he nonchalantly asked if she had ever considered having a little corrective surgery. Despite herself, Dana was shocked—she had no intention of letting Stephen make her over. Stephen backed off, but he was clearly displeased. Walking around a corner in the office the next day, Dana overheard a receptionist remark, "Looks like Cinderella is in for a little liposuction." She acted as if she hadn't heard it, but doubts had begun to creep in.

They had their first fight when Dana broke down and related the snide remark to Stephen, who got furious and threatened to fire the receptionist on the spot. "I don't think that's the point," Dana said. "I'm afraid you don't want me unless you get to turn me into someone I'm not." She knew all too well where her face and figure fell short of ideal, but how important was that to him? Stephen evaded the question and treated her coldly for the rest of the day. When Friday came, the night they usually spent together, he said he was too busy, but Dana got the distinct impression he was withholding sex to punish her.

The comparison to Cinderella was an apt one, but there was to be no fairy-tale ending. A week before they were to be married, Dana accidentally pressed the wrong phone button at the office, only to overhear Stephen talking to another woman. The tone of his voice and the subject of the conversation left no doubt that they were on intimate terms. Terribly hurt, Dana walked out of the office and never came back. She refused to take Stephen's calls, which quickly stopped. He protested that he still loved her, but Dana thought it sounded like an act to preserve his self-image. When he lamented how much money would be lost if they didn't go through with the ceremony, she burst into tears and hung up. Stephen never called again.

On the surface it would be difficult to imagine a courtship that came closer to the romantic ideal. Far more than most men, Stephen had the means and the desire to sweep a woman off her feet. He made Dana feel special and important, lavishing all his attention on her. But lovely as it seemed, this courtship had little to do with love and almost nothing to do with trust. What was really happening?

The key word here is *image*. Stephen was mainly interested in enhancing his self-image as a magician who could turn ordinary women into goddesses. Not only did he do this professionally but in personal relationships he had to be the star—he would probably have tried to "correct" the looks of the most beautiful woman on earth given the chance. His paying court, from the gifts to the sex, was a performance; Dana was quite right not to utter the slightest criticism of his sexual abilities, since he would have reacted badly. If they had gotten married, he would have lost interest in her and gone on to have affairs. One has only to note how completely he had excluded his first wife from his life to realize how much he needed new conquests to support his inflated self-image.

The only way Dana could have succeeded with Stephen would have been to allow herself to be bought; fortunately, her sense of self was based not on image but on her feelings. Being swept off her feet never felt quite real. Young as she was, she could tell that Stephen wasn't interested in connecting with her inner self and that he was even less interested in sharing his own.

In a way this story describes almost the perfect courtship—all we have to do is reverse everything that happened in it. A perfect courtship unfolds like a flower, as each partner becomes more comfortable exposing their inner world. It is a shared experience, with decisions made mutually and boundaries respected. One partner doesn't try to push the other beyond their boundaries, knowing that stretching a boundary is a gradual, delicate matter. The essence of courtship is communion, which this one totally lacked.

As hurt as she was, Dana was also secretly relieved that the wedding to Stephen didn't come off. Being turned into Cinderella had not fulfilled inner needs that I would call spiritual. Spiritually we all need things such as forgiveness, love, and compassion, but before any of these can be realized, we need to satisfy the most basic spiritual need: support on our path. You cannot expect another person to immediately understand your experiences as you enter into new and often confusing stages of spirituality, but if sharing is to take place, you must build a basis for satsang. This basis must include equality, sensitivity, and communication.

### Equality.

Being seen as equally important to your partner is a right many people cannot assert. Because we are all unequal in terms of intelligence, status, money, skills, and talents, these factors can become dominant in a relationship. A woman may feel, as Dana did, that the man who courts her has earned so many of life's advantages that she should be grateful for his success. The happiness she could expect in such a marriage, however, would have little spiritual validity.

In spirit everyone is equal. This isn't just an abstract concept; it is the one perception that can overcome ego. If I feel superior to you, my superiority is rooted in self-image. A self-image based upon money, for example, would make me think that I should be appreciated for all I have given you, which puts you at a disadvantage, since your own right to be appreciated doesn't have a comparable basis. When Stephen took Dana to an expensive restaurant, he put himself on a superior footing *in his eyes*. Thus he was protected from any criticism she might make, giving himself the right to say, "Look at what I'm providing. How can you be unhappy with me?"

Equality isn't based upon external factors or images. We all have an equal right to be appreciated, respected, and understood. Some men find it hard to extend this concept to a woman's emotions. They were not taught to value their own feelings, which get expressed only as a last resort. But to accept another person means accepting her emotions—there is nothing more basic or intrinsic. If this equality doesn't exist, how can spirit really grow? Spirit isn't an emotion, but it provides an opening to our inner selves. You have to feel that your partner wants to understand you and your feelings before you can share experiences you barely understand yourself.

### Sensitivity.

Being able to sense what is going on inside another person is a skill that has to be developed like any other. It isn't an easy one to acquire; you have to feel secure on the level of intuition, and you need to be able to accept complexity and conflicting emotions. The question "What are you feeling right now?" always has the answer "More than one thing." Sensitivity requires setting aside your notions of what the other person is feeling, what you think she should feel, and what you hope she isn't feeling. Whenever the ego intrudes, sensitivity cannot be present.

Sensitivity is easily crushed, but there is also social prejudice which holds that women are *too* sensitive (as men see it), and that sensitivity in a man makes him less masculine. Men therefore can find a ready excuse for shutting out others by claiming, "I don't understand why you feel this way" or "I don't have the slightest idea what's going on with you." If your mission in life is to protect your self-image, then opening up to another person's feelings runs contrary to your mission. To be sensitive you will have to abandon being right all the time, being in control, having needs that must dominate over the needs of others, and so forth.

In terms of Dana and Stephen, it was vital for Stephen *not* to be sensitive to any sign of discomfort from the woman he was wooing. He knew only one mode of courtship—Prince Charming sweeping Cinderella off her feet—and princes don't have flaws. If he sensed that Dana wasn't satisfied with his lavish generosity, he would have had to face the fact that everything he was doing was a performance. Most of us are made extremely uncomfortable by extreme generosity; it has a suffocating effect and makes the receiver feel inadequate compared with the giver. Dana felt all these things, but Stephen couldn't afford to be sensitive to them; he had no other way to "love" her, and to have allowed her to say how she wanted to be loved would have taken power out of his hands, which would have been intolerable.

### Communication.

*Communion* is the root word in *communication,* reminding us that to communicate with another person isn't to pass on information. It is to draw another into union with yourself. Women tend to have a more intuitive grasp of how communication works, for both positive and negative reasons. On the positive side girls are typically taught from a young age to value bonding, especially on an emotional level, whereas boys are typically taught to compete. In a competitive situation, silence is often equated with power. On the negative side, women often don't expect to have power; therefore, they can "afford" to expose their feelings and inner conflicts. By contrast, if a man in power communicates too much of his inner fears, insecurities, or conflicts, his right to power may be questioned.

These social expectations have a large influence on relationships. A man may sincerely feel that he has nothing to say about his feelings, and conversely that women don't talk reasonably about situations. A woman may feel "stupid" when what she has to say is consistently emotional, and she may conversely feel that the absence of emotional communication from men means that they are stronger. In Dana's story, communication was confined by the rules of the Cinderella fairy tale. Dana couldn't easily express anything outside the boundaries of the story of a working woman meeting a prince and being carried off by him to great heights of wealth and power. Stephen's vision of what was going on took precedence over her perceptions, reflecting both a breakdown in communication and a loss of equality.

By the time two people are married, they both know the limits of what to expect from each other in terms of equality, sensitivity, and communication. By establishing these factors in the courtship phase, you find out what you are getting into before limits are drawn.

If you find yourself in a long-standing relationship, think back to your courtship days. Ask yourself what you wanted from a mate back then and compare it with what you have. Inevitably you will find that equality is something you both can work on, sensitivity can always be made deeper, and communication must be worked at every day. Keeping these alive is the basis for spiritual growth together, whether you have only just emerged from infatuation or have been married for years.

# INTIMACY:
## THE INNOCENCE OF DESIRE

The issue hovering over intimacy, the next phase of romance, is desire. Desire is a driving force behind love, but it isn't the same as love, and where the two diverge, many conflicts arise. The ancient Sanskrit word for desire is *Kama,* made famous by the book of erotic lore called *Kama Sutra,* the "teaching about desire." But *Kama* is a much broader term; it applies to desires or wishes of every kind.

A formula I learned in my childhood in India, inherited from the ancient scriptures, holds that life is perfected by achieving four things: Artha, Kama, Dharma, and Moksha. Artha is wealth, kama is the fulfillment of one's desires, dharma is right livelihood or work, and moksha is the liberation of the soul.

On the path to love, all four aims of life get fulfilled, and this is where issues arise, since it is still difficult for many people to accept that desire is legitimate. Desire remains tainted with implications of selfishness and "lower" drives. The one place in our lives where most of us feel free to express kama is romance. The erotic longing that is part of romantic love inspires every lover to merge with the beloved; this is the natural consummation of attraction between two people.

The great Bengali poet Rabindranath Tagore wrote delicately erotic verses in his adolescence, and one says,

> Leaving their homes, two loves have made
> a pilgrimage to the confluence of lips.
> In the law of Love, two waves have swelled,
> breaking and mingling on two lips.

This may seem like a chaste poem comparing two lovers to religious devotees making their way, as Indian pilgrims are wont to do, to the sacred confluence of two holy rivers. If you understand Tagore's original Bengali, however, you would know that the word for confluence is the same as the word for the act of making love. Now the poem seems almost sacrilegious, when in fact it is an unembarrassed blending of flesh and spirit. In the West we might say that the sacred has met the profane, except that to Tagore, and for anyone who has fallen deeply in love, the profane *is* sacred.

The insights of the intimacy phase pertain to the union of flesh and spirit:

*Fulfillment is natural and not to be ashamed of.*

*Ecstasy is a state of the soul transmitted through the body.*

*Union consists of two people opening to the same Being.*

These insights are based on approaching desire without guilt or inhibition. In traditional cultures, however, sexual consummation wasn't permitted immediately after two people fell passionately in love, out of a belief that desire should be postponed. There were many reasons for imposing a waiting period, but one was the belief that love and desire are not compatible. Either desire is of the flesh and therefore sinful or else it is a prize not to be given by a woman until the union is signed and sealed through marriage.

Today, in modern society, the consummation of desire comes early, awaiting nothing but the consent of a man and a woman. Courtship is not nearly as bound by convention as in the past; it can be as long or as short as two people want. However, this doesn't mean that the issue of desire has been resolved. Emotional residues linger from the traditional view, which by holding out a woman's virginity as a sacred prize had a built-in conflict. You cannot say that desire is sinful while at the same time holding out sexual fulfillment as a prize. Why would love ever accept a sin as its prize?

Traditional religious teaching has blinded us to the fact that flesh and spirit are two poles that belong together. Romantic love is undeniably sexual; yet it contains the potential for great spiritual experiences. The beauty of sensuality has its own spiritual significance without resort to "higher" values. An ancient Sanskrit text exults in the joy of intimacy:

> When we have loved, my love,
>   Panting and pale from love,
> Then from your cheeks, my love,
>   Scent of the sweat I love:
> And when our bodies love
>   Now to relax in love
> After the stress of love,
>   Ever still more I love
> Our mingled breath of love.

The frankness of this declaration of passion is refreshing, for it reminds us that the spiritual union of lovers isn't separate from the sweat and mingled breath of sexuality.

*Sex allows you to blend the needs of the self with the freedom of the Self.*

The word *kama* is used to describe not just sexual desire but the desire to be united with God. By implication this is the same kama that makes you want to be united with your Self. If you could listen to the voice of spirit at every moment, you would hear that your divine nature longs for you as you long for it.

## A NEW INTIMACY:
## INTIMACY WITH THE SELF

What raises romantic love above lesser pleasures is that it stirs our deep erotic natures. This is yet another source of anxiety for modern people, who are obsessed by sex without being willing to lose control, without being able to surrender to real passion.

*Passion must contain surrender in order to be authentic.*

But surrender to what? To the convergence of all the aspects of your being that need to flow into the erotic moment. Physical sensuality, spiritual ecstasy, erotic flowering—when all these converge, the sexual act becomes sacred, and what is sacred contains the deepest pleasure. Thousands of years ago, Lord Shiva murmured to his consort, "While being caressed, sweet princess, enter the caress as everlasting life." This remains the ideal of intimacy.

Because intimacy is now so totally identified with the sexual act, fulfillment has become confused with performance. Orgasm is pursued with a devotion that would put most religious zealots to shame. The assumption for a long time was that men are most anxious about their ability to perform, but now that nonorgasmic women have become more frank and open about their predicament, it appears that the anxiety is fully shared.

Intimacy in the physical sense is usually taken to be the same as having an orgasm. But no matter how exciting it is, an orgasm is a sensation centered in the ego. True intimacy is shared self-expression.

For a man to be intimate with a woman, both have to be able to release themselves into the special state that orgasm brings, even though they cannot literally share the same sensations. Orgasm isn't a fixed thing. For some people it is a release, for others an opening, for still others a contraction. In all cases, though, there is a shift of experience that is not only pleasurable but in some way deeply transforming. Spiritual masters tell us that the state of enlightenment, which is totally free, ecstatic, and unbounded, is glimpsed very closely in orgasm. Or at least this is its potential.

Although there is a certain loss when intimacy is entered hastily, our present approach to sexuality has the advantage of removing outworn taboos. More than any time in the past, couples today are experiencing sexuality frankly and openly before making a commitment to proceed further in their relationship. Desire isn't so highly prized anymore, yet its spiritual potential remains intact.

When two people become physically intimate, they do not necessarily become united. Physical union can coexist with separateness, because for both partners the ego can remain involved. The ideal of stepping into shared ecstasy isn't reached by practicing some technique that raises orgasm to the heights of bliss. Having sex with another person is really just one way to make an agreement. The agreement may be serious or trivial; it may betoken a deep commitment or little more than a passing encounter.

To see intimacy as an agreement is a very healthy thing, because otherwise the sexual act becomes entangled in hidden agendas. Fantasy is never more powerful or more misleading than where sex is concerned. For a woman the hidden agenda often takes the form of believing that having sex equals love. A man's hidden agenda is more likely to equate sex with power. This was particularly true in times when the man was the pursuer, ardently offering his love, which the woman would reject or accept. The ultimate token of acceptance was for her to "give in" to the sexual act. In doing so she accepted love at the same time. Many women still harbor this belief in fantasy form.

For his part, the man knew that sexual surrender meant that his pursuit had been successful; the hunter had struck his mark at the same moment that the lover was embraced. In the past it seemed only natural for both sexes to use the aggressive image of the hunt as symbolic of the quest for intimacy, yet looking back we can see a good deal of hidden fear and insecurity in this analogy. Why should the act of love be linked to aggression at all?

These symbols and images were part of a social code, therefore they required no agreement. It wasn't possible for either men or women to exempt themselves from the code. Today the opposite is true. If a man feels himself to be a hunter, conqueror, or ardent pursuer, that is his own choice. If a woman sees herself as prey, prize, or unattainable love object, that is her decision. No single code operates anymore, and by making intimacy an agreement, both parties can approach sexuality openly as something they mutually want. Having sex with someone else does not imply that you have entered his belief system or will fulfill her expectations. You are not implicitly playing a part in his fantasy or expecting your version of love to match hers.

But there is a price to pay. In many ways sexual freedom is frightening because of the loss of boundaries. The old social code linked love and sex. For a woman to believe that a man loved her because he desired her was unchallenged. For a man to believe that having sex secured a woman's love was just as natural. Now that this is a matter of agreement, it can also be a cause of disagreement. Love and desire are essentially separate, a matter open for discussion.

It is surprising how many people enter sexual intimacy with no idea of what they are agreeing to. It is still common for both men and women to bring expectations to bed. Because these expectations are founded on images from the past, they defeat the possibility of passionate surrender. You cannot surrender to an image but can only play it out, and the more often you play it out, the less spontaneous sex becomes.

To rob sex of its spontaneity makes it both false and ugly. Sexuality is the most spontaneous aspect of our lives. It is the one place where we do not have to put at risk our abilities, intellect, and social personae. Playing a part is a necessity none of us can completely escape in everyday life. We all have roles as workers, family members, citizens, and so forth. Undeniably this places strain upon many other urges that would like to gain expression but are not permitted to do so. You cannot give way to every impulse of anger at work, much less walk out at will. You cannot decide to stop supporting a family on a whim, since the very fabric of society depends upon bearing one's share of responsibility.

Duty hems in desire at every turn, to the point that most people come to believe that suppressing their desires, holding themselves in check, is good. Suppression is not good, however; it is only expedient. Society requires that we draw limits on the expression of desire, which makes it all the more necessary to have at least one area of life that is completely free and uninhibited. Intimacy is meant to be just such an area. What is it that makes sex free or inhibited, loving or merely pleasurable?

## FREEDOM AND INTIMACY

Many people deny themselves free, loving sex—even if they are not aware of doing so—because they approach the sexual act in terms of results. They assume that any orgasm is good, and a good orgasm is better. Not only do we evaluate whether sex was "successful" but we hold up physical pleasure as the primary goal. Pleasure is a natural thing but it is also an elusive one. For some people the pleasure of sex is that it promises a release for anxiety and stress. For them "success" is actually negative, being defined as the escape from tension.

Other ingredients can be mixed into the sexual act that are far from loving. Someone who has bottled-up rage inside will usually make love in a way that is overly aggressive or competitive. A fearful person will typically find it difficult to allow anything like a full release into bodily sensations; his or her holding back is a passive way to act out fear and at the same time miss any encounter with love.

There are many variations on this theme, for as much as we would wish to be good lovers, we all bring our conflicts and needs to bed. Whatever blocks our pleasure also blocks love, because in sex pleasure is the doorway to love.

Even though sex is meant to be uninhibited and free, there are always degrees of freedom. Rarely do we believe that we deserve pleasure without limits. How, then, can we give love without limits, or receive it?

Rather than examining the results of the sexual act, we need to consider its beginnings. Intimacy starts not with a physical approach but with a set of beliefs. The primary beliefs that defeat pleasure include the following:

> Sex is too powerful and has to be controlled.
> Sin is attached to sex, making it guilty and shameful.
> Asking someone else to give you pleasure is greedy and
>   selfish.
> Surrendering to pleasure is the same as surrendering your
>   power.

What all of these beliefs have in common is that they provide a reason to suppress desire.

*When sex is deprived of its spiritual connection, some aspect of desire is being suppressed.*

The spiritual dimension of sex is its joyfulness and ecstasy, its communication of love between two people. These qualities do not require effort; they appear spontaneously when sex itself is spontaneous. However, a great deal of spiritual teaching has been openly antisexual. As long as the credo "It is better to marry than to burn" was in effect, spiritual value was assigned not to intimacy but to chastity. When spiritual teachers held up chastity as a virtue—as they have in every tradition East and West—the intention was not to make pleasure a sin but to elevate a higher virtue that by implication led to higher pleasure. One feels the truth in Krishnamurti's words, "Trying to suppress sexual urges is a form of ugliness that in itself cannot be chaste. Chastity of the monk with his vows is worldliness as long as the urges are present. All walls of separateness turn life into a battlefield."

Chastity in the sense of purity is a spiritual good, but it should not be mistaken for suppression of desire. When he asks why people try to repress their desires, Krishnamurti makes the following beautiful argument: resisting the sexual urge has been held up as something good to do, but if we look at it, resistance is born of fear. We are afraid of being wrong, of stepping out of line. Society, anxious to make us conform, tells us that if we don't resist our sexual urges, we will go out of control.

Yet is this really true? If sex is natural, why does it have to be controlled? In fact the whole conflict over sex, the problems of neurosis and deviancy, and sexual misbehavior, can be traced to resistance, not to sexual urges. Resistance is always mental; it implies a judgment against what is actually being felt. Sex becomes a problem when it gets mixed with hidden emotions such as shame, anger, and guilt. Under those circumstances the sexual impulse is confusing. When people ask questions like "Is it all right to have sex with anyone you want to?" or "Is it natural to be monogamous?" the implication is that an outside judgment must enter into the issue.

Values are personal; each situation that has sexual energy in it involves the whole human being. If you understand where you are in a sexual situation—meaning that your emotions and values are in your awareness with clarity—the sexual drive doesn't stand apart like a raging intruder. It is part of you; it is acceptable and loved.

If you can walk through life without resistance, you will discover that life in itself is chaste. It has a purity that includes both love and sex—there is no division between them except in society's misguided conditioning.

This argument has a very deep spiritual basis. Most of the time our worries over sex involve thinking and talking about it, yet sex isn't a word or a thought. It isn't divided in any way from the flow of life; its urge arises, asks for fulfillment, and disappears without leaving traces of guilt and shame unless we add those traces by our beliefs. If sex gets tied down to the mere pursuit of pleasure, it will result in pain, for pleasure cannot be kept up forever; it will lead only to meaningless repetition and frustration, to a compulsive craving for sensations that can only dwindle in satisfaction.

As Krishnamurti says, the mere pursuit of pleasure throws life out the window. By "life" he means the sacred Being at the heart of existence, the mystery that can be known only by not resisting, by being natural. The difference between sex, love, and chastity doesn't exist; they are one.

In a world where imitating other people's ideas and values is forced on us in thousands of ways, sex is left as a means of escaping ourselves. It is a form of self-forgetfulness that is many people's only real form of meditation. Such is the promise of intimacy that it can deliver us into a place where experience of the spirit is genuine and undeniable.

# LOVING PRACTICE

## Freeing Sexual Blocks

If you want to improve your sexual experiences, the last place to start with is practice in the bedroom. Sex is naturally spontaneous; it is both expression and release, excitement and relaxation. The best sex is the most open and unplanned; therefore planning for the unplanned is more or less a self-contradiction. There is no way to practice being spontaneous.

> To improve your sexual experience, first get rid of your expectations.

Sexual energy is neutral; you can associate it with anything, positive or negative, in your life. Whatever you expect sex to be, it will tend to become. So-called sexual problems are actually ingrained behaviors that block the free flow of sexual energy. In both men and women the physiology of sex is very delicate and easily influenced by the mind. It is your mind that judges "good" and "bad" sex; it is your mind that intervenes to prevent orgasm or potency (leaving aside disease conditions that impose physical limitations).

The dilemma is that coming to bed without expectations seems to be impossible, given how the mind works. When sexual experience was new, it contained a quality of surprise and innocence. Even

142

if we cannot remember our first orgasm, most of us can remember how different orgasm was from other pleasurable sensations. Its newness and intensity caused us to want more, but as you repeat any sensation, it becomes familiar, and familiarity leads to dullness. For many people sex becomes associated with performance. The question "How well am I doing?" hovers over the bedroom. For other people sex is associated with sensation. The question "How am I feeling?" is uppermost in their minds. And for still others, security is dominant; the question "Do you really love me?" is in their minds while making love.

As soon as sex becomes bound up in these secondary associations and needs, it is no longer free. There is nothing bad about pursuing unrelated needs in sex. Orgasm is a psychological package, not a physical reflex. But no matter how well you perform or how terrific you feel, laying orgasm into a certain groove separates it from any spiritual significance.

*Sex is mechanical when it is without spiritual meaning.*

For many reasons, it is difficult to align our sexual and spiritual natures. The following exercise is aimed not at making sex more spiritual but at removing the obstacles that prevent spirit from entering into it.

## PART ONE

Look at the following list of statements and write "Agree" or "Disagree" beside each. Be honest and keep in mind that having expectations isn't something to feel bad about—this is an exercise in self-knowledge.

1. Sex is better if it lasts a long time.

2. Orgasm should be intense.

3. It's not sex without orgasm.

4. I'm pretty insistent on getting sex when I want it.

5. The more orgasms, the better.

6. The best sex I ever had wasn't with my present partner.

7. Impotence lets my partner down.

*or*

Not having an orgasm lets my partner down.

8. My partner isn't as open about new positions and techniques as I am.

9. I've gone along with sexual experiments I didn't feel comfortable with just because my partner asked me to.

10. I aim to please. I rarely let my partner down.

11. My partner disappoints me a lot more often than he (or she) knows.

12. I wouldn't like anyone to think I get too carried away over sex.

13. I'm too embarrassed to discuss some of the things I'd like to do in bed.

14. We have sex more (or less) often than I'd like.

15. I miss the way our sex used to be.

16. I really don't think about sex that often.

17. Our sex isn't so great, but the rest of our marriage makes up for that.

18. I have fantasies I don't share with my partner.

19. My mind wanders during sex.

20. I'm not such a great lover.

These very common statements indicate that everyone has less than healthy sexual expectations at least some of the time.

➤ *If you agreed with five statements or fewer,* you are likely to be very present with your sexuality and appreciative of sex as it is happening. You don't have many fixed expectations or adherence to values outside yourself.

➤ *If you agreed with six or more statements,* you are bringing issues to bed that are interfering with the free flow of sexual energy—your sex is beset by ego concerns and expectations.

➤ *If you agreed with none of the statements,* either you are a highly evolved lover or you haven't answered as honestly as you could.

Now let's discuss how you felt while reading these statements. Some are much more likely to trigger emotional charges than others. Reread the list and check your emotional reactions. Do you feel very uncomfortable reading certain sentences? Do you feel nothing? To be at either extreme implies that sexual energy is being held inside—any repressed feeling keeps sexual energy from flowing. Among the most powerful sexual blocks are shame, guilt, doubt, discouragement, and embarrassment.

If you feel strong emotion over "I'm not such a great lover," for example, it's not difficult to see that lack of self-worth is an issue. Someone who strongly agrees with "I aim to please. I rarely let my partner down" is equally prey to self-doubt, only less consciously. If you probe your feelings of discomfort and release them, you will do more for your sex life than if you focus on the mechanics of sex.

You can release your sexual blocks in the following way:

1. Pick a statement that you feel strongly about, either positively or negatively.
2. Lie down, take a deep breath, and let yourself feel what is going on when you think about the statement.
3. Ask to be guided to the meaning of the statement. If nothing comes to mind, ask for blocks to be removed. A helpful technique here is to pant in quick, shallow breaths—this distracts the mind from holding on to its blocks.

4. When you have some kind of answer—an image, an insight, a strong wave of feeling—ask for release. Take a deep breath and let go of whatever wants to come out: a sob, a scream, physical movement, a deep sigh, or simply a wave of fatigue.

5. Relive any memories that want to surface.

6. When you feel that you are fully in touch with the emotional charge behind the statement, ask for a clearing of the charge. Breathe evenly until you relax and any tension associated with the statement has been released.

*When blocks are removed, sexual energy has no choice but to flow.*

Each statement in the questionnaire has a wide range of possible meanings that may or may not apply to you, but here are the types of blocks generally indicated:

1. *Sex is better if it lasts a long time.*
   Fixed expectations from sex, comparison with others, social norms more important than personal experience

2. *Orgasm should be intense.*
   Comparison with the past, valuing of physical sensation over emotions, self-absorption, addictive personality traits

3. *It's not sex without orgasm.*
   Performance anxiety, comparison with past, valuing of physical sensation over emotions

4. *I'm pretty insistent on getting sex when I want it.*
   Hidden anger or sadism, self-absorption, competitiveness

5. *The more orgasms, the better.*
   Performance fixation, wandering attention (counting instead of being present), comparison with social norms, emotional immaturity

6. *The best sex I ever had wasn't with my present partner.*
   Disappointment, anger toward partner, discouragement, inability to be present

7. *Impotence lets my partner down.*

   or

   *Not having an orgasm lets my partner down.*
   Performance anxiety, low self-worth, inhibited physical release, hidden anger

8. *My partner isn't as open about new positions and techniques as I am.*
   Lack of communication, fixation on fantasy or sensations, judgment against partner

9. *I've gone along with sexual experiments I didn't feel comfortable with just because my partner asked me to.*
   Overdependence, low self-worth, lack of communication

10. *I aim to please. I rarely let my partner down.*
    Performance anxiety hidden by performance success, self-absorption, competitiveness

11. *My partner disappoints me a lot more often than he (or she) knows.*
    Overdependence, low self-worth, abuse background, detachment from sexual drive

12. *I wouldn't like anyone to think I get too carried away over sex.*
    Valuing of social norms over personal satisfaction, detachment from sexual desire, low self-worth

13. *I'm too embarrassed to discuss some of the things I'd like to do in bed.*
    Fixation on fantasy, distrust of partner, negative judgments against sex from parents

14. *We have sex more (or less) often than I'd like.*
    Overdependence, low self-worth, lack of communication

15. *I miss the way our sex used to be.*
    Lack of communication, outside distractions, estrangement from partner

16. *I really don't think about sex that often.*
    Disappointment or anger toward partner, low self-image, judgment against sexual drive

17. *Our sex isn't so great, but the rest of our marriage makes up for that.*
    Inertia, lack of attention to sex, distractions from intimacy

18. *I have fantasies I don't share with my partner.*
    Lack of communication, fear of sexual drive, abuse background, distrust

19. *My mind wanders during sex.*
    Inhibition, disappointment or anger toward partner, distraction from sexual drive, high stress

20. *I'm not such a great lover.*
    Overdependence, wounded self-image, sexual trauma in the past, judgment against sex

These are very general interpretations in what is a wide spectrum of possibilities. To feel that you aren't a great lover, for example, can be a sign of something mild, such as sexual inexperience, or something severe, such as clinical depression. Rather than reading any of these characterizations as a diagnosis or judgment, see if they show the way to hidden issues you may not be facing. The point is not to make you feel that there is something wrong with you, only to stir energies that need to move.

## PART TWO

In our culture "good sex" is usually defined in terms of technique and performance. We overlook that sex is a creative act, which doesn't need to be critiqued or evaluated. Biologically, human sexuality is essential to the process that creates babies, but the same energy contributes to many things at levels of life that are not literally biological. Sex is creativity itself, and we have the capacity to create on every plane of existence, from the biological to the spiritual.

Sex is creative when it produces a new feeling, insight, or experience. In this exercise some of these possibilities are explored.

Look at the following list of experiences. Put a check by any you have had at least once during sex. These are suggestive phrases, to be interpreted as you wish—your own perception of bliss, carefreeness, playfulness, and so on is all you need to go by.

Delighted laughter
Sense of timelessness
Ecstasy
Warm flow in the heart
Merging with partner
Floating sensation, as if the body disappears
Warmth or visible light flowing up the spine
Loss of ego
Carefreeness
Playfulness

Nonattachment to your performance

Complete letting go

Expansion

Sense of wholeness, safety, belonging

Blessing

Bliss

Acute awareness of self or surroundings

Unbounded love

Contentment, peace in the center of your heart

Now look back over your answers; the experiences you have checked indicate your spiritual horizon. That is, you have learned to use sexual energy to create these experiences. If you have some only once, these are the envelope of your inner growth. The experiences you have had more than once, especially if recently, indicate the growth you have already integrated into your loving personality.

Go back over the list and mark experiences you haven't had but think could happen next. These are your spiritual goals. Your desire for them is enough to bring them about; on your inner landscape you are already working toward them.

Now go through the list a third time and mark the experiences you believe are out of reach or impossible for you. These could be interpreted as blocks to spirit. Since nothing is truly out of reach in the creative use of sexuality, naming what you see as "impossible" experiences holds up a mirror to your current belief in the limits of love.

On the path to love impossibilities are resolved by turning non-love into love. With spiritual growth comes new creative potential—which can take the form of sexual expression—leading to the realization that you are pure potential, able to fulfill any creative impulse.

# In Our Lives

## The Worn-out Lover

For a long time, ever since his early teens, Guy had been a lover, and a very active one. The singles bar scene had been his second home for a decade, and he considered himself a born appreciator of women, unable to comprehend why other men seemed to resent or ignore them. To Guy women were intoxicating creatures, and giving them pleasure was something he felt proud of. He never called himself a woman's boyfriend; he was always her lover. He took the sexual revolution for granted—he was open to almost any sexual experiment proposed by the women he dated, and he could quickly take his partner to a place where she wasn't embarrassed to express her fantasies.

When asked how he felt about his many conquests, Guy said, "I loved every one of them. Nothing makes me happier than a grateful woman." He was sincere when he claimed that none of his former flames resented him in any way, despite the fact that his liaisons with them lasted only a few nights or a few months—six at most.

Caroline was the first woman Guy had ever met whom he did not want to take to bed immediately, despite the fact that he was strongly attracted to her. She was in her early twenties—Guy was about to turn thirty—but she radiated the demure, innocent quality of a much younger girl. Enchanted, Guy thought of Caroline as a fawn, with her large, trusting eyes and slight air of aloofness.

For her part, Caroline seemed to adore Guy; he was only her third serious boyfriend (she definitely preferred this term over *lover*). Shaking off his reluctance, Guy soon entered an intimate relationship with Caroline. All went smoothly until one night when he found himself, quite unexpectedly, waking up in tears at two in the morning. An uncontrollable emotion—was it grief? remorse?—swept over him. Mystified and shaken, Guy went back to sleep.

The next time he took Caroline to bed, however, Guy found himself performing far below his usual high standards. His mind wandered, and for the first time he felt that he might not be able to reach orgasm. This impossibility wasn't allowed to happen, but afterward he felt fatigued and joyless. Caroline made no comment; she held Guy for a long time before he fell asleep.

Their relationship deepened. In many ways Guy felt that he was going through the happiest time of his life. Caroline's light heart and innocent manner came as a revelation to him; he sometimes felt by comparison that he had been working very hard at life. This was undoubtedly true in his career—Guy worked long hours creating databases for a prestigious commercial realtor. His goal was to be a millionaire in five years. Caroline was the first woman who had ever distracted him from this ambition.

When Guy decided to propose to her, his ears burned in disbelief as Caroline asked for a little more time. Disbelief turned to shock when she hesitantly said that she wanted their relationship not to be intimate for a while. Pressed for reasons, Caroline hesitated even more, but finally she half-whispered, "I don't think you really like it. You just don't want to let me down."

It was the most troubling and yet the most honest thing a woman had ever said to Guy. That night he stormed out in hurt pride, but he knew in his heart that he felt worn out. Certain things about sex had never occurred to him. For instance, he had never thought that more isn't necessarily better. For ten years he'd had sex nearly every day, and the need behind this obsession struck him now as something like addiction. It had also never occurred to him that other voices could speak during the act of sex. He had obeyed the voice of desire so completely that now he found it difficult to hear expressions of sadness, pent-up anger, and grief. Reflecting on it, he realized they must always have been present.

When Guy came back to Caroline, he loved her enough to be able to thank her for having proposed a waiting period. The two started to reconstruct a sexual relationship, beginning with simple touch. They would lie together and easily ask each other for a gentle touch on some part of their bodies, directing where to touch next, how long to stay in one place.

Rather than finding this erotic, Guy often discovered that some touches aroused anxiety; at times he felt like crying. Gradually he realized that feeling safe with women had been rare for him, and that because he felt safe with Caroline, old wounds could be released. He found that as pent-up emotions began to surface, he wanted to tell Caroline about incidents from his past that he had never shared with a woman—in fact, talking to women had never been his strong suit. He began to make links between his need to perform in bed and his demanding, critical mother. In time it became clear to him that at some level he felt all women were demanding, and by being a skillful lover he could defuse in advance their contempt for him as inadequate.

Guy was fortunate that so much love remained in him—many men could have taken a decade to achieve the insight he was gaining in a few months. Caroline did not set herself up as teacher or therapist; she followed Guy in his self-discovery, allowing him to withdraw when he needed to. It became clear to him that she had given herself permission to withdraw as well. To him having sex had always been a sign of intimacy; for Caroline intimacy emerged slowly, and agreeing to have sex with him had been only a first step.

Some hard times followed for Guy. There were nights when he felt aggressive or angry during sex, which led to deep bouts of guilt. His image of himself as "lover" frayed as he came to feel the underlying rage he had suppressed, compelling him to act out sexually what he idealized as his inner personality. He wasn't the sensitive, generous, caring lover he had fashioned himself into but a complex, and sometimes contradictory, bundle of feelings and drives. In time this was good enough, since it was real.

Caroline realized that it was important to support Guy in his spiritual progress; as it turned out she was quite serious about her own spiritual life, so she was able to view this transition as more than psychological. She believed that all the changes in their relationship were serving to bring Guy and her into unity. To help chart their progress, she made a list of experiences she wanted to have with Guy, noticing each one and discussing it with him as each occurred.

> I want to feel needed for who I am.
> I want to feel vulnerable.
> I want to feel you won't ever hurt me.
> I want to feel your strength.
> I want to feel I can tell you what I most desire.
> I want to feel open.
> I want to feel a gentle wildness.
> I want to feel one with you.
> I want to feel nothing was ever better than this.
> I want to feel lightness bubbling in my heart.
> I want to feel profound.
> I want to feel at one.

This was more than a wish list; it sent a message of desire to the universe that she expected to be fulfilled as events unfolded. Caroline encouraged Guy to make his own list. They didn't bring these lists to bed or think about them while in bed. The point was to articulate clearly where they wanted their path together to lead.

Marriage came a year later, by which time Guy had changed many of his most basic attitudes toward sex. He no longer performed it without love, and he felt able to say when his emotions made love difficult. He thought not of sexual excitement but of being comfortable. He found that the strongest turn-ons were silent, peaceful surroundings, tender expressions, deep looks of desire, sparkling eyes, tentative touches, and modesty. There were moments when he forgot about sex, lost in the sheer freedom and openness of his own being, and these were the most sexual moments of all. For someone who had spent his growing-up years drowned in sexual experience, Guy was on his way to recovering the one thing experience cannot bring—the freedom of innocence.

# 4

# HOW TO SURRENDER

—🍃—

Spiritually, no action is more important than surrender. Surrender is the tenderest impulse of the heart, acting out of love to give whatever the beloved wants. Surrender is being alert to exactly what is happening now, not imposing expectations from the past. Surrender is faith that the power of love can accomplish anything, even when you cannot foresee the outcome of a situation.

But surrendering to another person's ego, even your beloved's, is not a spiritual act. There is a deeper, more mystical meaning to surrender. At the level of ego, two people cannot want exactly the same thing all the time. Yet at the level of spirit, they cannot help but want the same thing all the time. Your ego wants material things, predictable conclusions, continuity, security, and the prerogative to be right when others are wrong. By definition, pursuing these goals shuts out another person unless she falls in line with "my" agenda or he realizes that "I" am the important one around here.

Your spirit is not involved in such concerns. It wants being, love, freedom, and creative opportunities. This is an entirely different level of desire, and when you reach it you can share yourself with another person without conflict. Such sharing is the core of surrender.

Most people are raised to pursue ego goals, often without question. The choice to remain on this level is always open. But you also have the choice to move onto the plane of spirit, with its very different goals. The gap between ego and spirit is unavoidable. It would seem impossible to close this gap, since spirit and ego are total opposites. Bringing them together is achieved through surrender, and the only force that can accomplish it is love. Surrender, then, is the next phase on love's journey, which you enter as soon as you choose to be in relationship.

The majority of people find themselves not in romance but in a long-term relationship, usually marriage. This phase occupies much more of our lives than falling in love ever could. If falling in love is a brief opening to spirit, long-term relationship is the broad plateau that follows—we will simply call this plateau commitment. Commitment is extremely difficult for many people, and countless psychological reasons have been given for why this is so. But the spiritual difficulty of commitment is that it throws you directly into the gap between ego and spirit. Each person brings into a marriage a complex bundle of ego needs; the husband may be loving and kind, but his ego demands that life turn out according to certain expectations, and the same may be true for the wife. A relationship based on need is not love. Either the two egos must live in an uneasy truce or they must find another way—surrender.

Throughout the earlier phase of romance there has been a sense of being chosen, as if an irresistible force has invaded your heart, but in relationship the path to love is not automatic. One must choose, day to day, to stay on it. Rather than seeing surrender in terms of another person, we should call it surrender to the path. The insights that arise in a committed relationship therefore are those pertaining to the path:

> *You are on a unique path created between you and your beloved.*
>
> *You find your path not by thinking, feeling, or doing but by surrendering.*
>
> *Surrender reveals the impulses of spirit beneath the mask of ego.*

The path to love uses relationship to move you out of your limited sense of "I," "me," "mine" into an expanded identity—this is the growth from self to Self.

## DHARMA IN LOVE

There is a fundamental mystery to the soul, that its integrity is not violated by merging with another person. The blending of two spirits brings more to the union than each partner started with. The process of soul-making that used to be for "me" is now for "us." Rumi expresses this beautifully in a few heartfelt words:

> My soul glowed from the fire of your fire.
> Your world was a whispering water
> At the river of my heart.

The realization that two can be as one is the essence of surrender; if marriage were just the conjunction of two people who never departed from the walled camp of their isolation, human existence would not be able to scale the spiritual heights. And yet it does.

Although they may not admit it, most people secretly mourn the transition from romance to commitment. Being in a relationship, since it requires patience, devotion, and persistence, is much more difficult than falling in love. Its spiritual rewards are won through dedication to inner growth. What this implies to many people is work. Romance is recess, relationship is school. Because it is hard, marriage often dwindles in passion; it brings conflict, disappointment, and pain. It can result in total mistrust and betrayal if it ends badly. Yet this whole story is an ego story.

The only real difference between romance and relationship, spiritually speaking, has to do with surrender. Surrender comes naturally to two people when they first fall in love. Being lost in the deliciousness of romance, they have no time to be selfish, no will to distrust. Marriage doesn't proceed on that basis. The mask of fantasy is stripped away once two people have engaged in intimacy over a period of time, and the grace period of selflessness is up. The ego returns with a vengeance, insisting on "my" needs; therefore, surrender has to become a conscious goal—it is no longer a given. This isn't to say that surrender is hard work; it is *conscious* work. As such it can bring the same joy and delight as falling in love, the same sense of play that releases new lovers from their ego burdens.

> *Making your relationship as extraordinary as falling in love*
> *is the great challenge of this stage.*

In one of his poems D. H. Lawrence speaks of passionate romantic love as being like a flower while marriage is like a hard gem that endures.

> That is the crystal of peace, the slow hard jewel of trust,
>   the sapphire of fidelity.

159

The gem of mutual peace emerging from the wild chaos of
love.

Why should you be committed to someone else? Peace, fidelity,
trust—the key words are given in these few verses. The most profound reason for committing to another person is also the simplest:
marriage is sacred. When they are fully committed in love, the husband sees God in the wife and the wife sees God in the husband.
On this basis they are able to surrender to each other, because they
are only surrendering to the spirit in everything.

These words sound almost shocking in a modern context. Surrender is a remote possibility in relationships today. Most marriages
struggle just to establish basic personal trust. Psychologists hold that
the first ten years of a marriage are spent resolving differences of
thought, habit, ways of doing things, likes and dislikes. "I want
orange juice in the morning, but you bought apple juice." "I prefer
the right side of the bed, but so do you." "This color isn't right for
the living room, even if you do like it." The magnificence of a sacred
relationship crashes on the rocks of trivial ego conflicts.

In all this chaos the spiritual meaning of marriage has become as
diffuse as the meaning of love itself. Is commitment worth it anymore? Can surrender be possible amid so much battering conflict? If
you set aside the present social context for a moment, a sacred
marriage, in which both partners surrender to each other as expressions of spirit, is natural. It is the ripening of love's fruit after the
blossoming of romance.

*Romance is a temporary state of the sacred. Relationship
makes it permanent.*

The ancient Indian word *Dharma* describes much more completely what I mean by "sacred." The noun *dharma* comes from the root verb meaning "to sustain or uphold," and like many words in Sanskrit, this one has layers of meaning. Whatever upholds a person's life and keeps it on a proper course is considered dharmic. It is dharmic to tell the truth and not to lie, or to be faithful in marriage instead of straying.

*Dharma* is also translated as "law" or "righteousness." In India today someone who follows the family tradition of work, worship, and social behavior is also said to be in his dharma. Modern Western society is not dharmic in any of these ways, since our children feel free to choose very different occupations from their parents', along with new codes of behavior and new places to live. In both East and West the rootedness of a dharmic society has been undermined in this century.

However, dharma is more than a social convention; it is a living force that can bring you through the many threats and challenges of life. Your ego does not believe this, for it cannot find dharma; ego is not guided by love, and dharma is intimately tied to love. In the West the closest concept to dharma is grace, the loving presence of God that keeps humanity under divine protection. When Jesus spoke of God seeing the fall of a sparrow, he was referring to dharma. In China the same concept emerged as *Tao*, or "the Way," which was seen as an invisible but real power that organizes all life. Being in tune with "the Way" is the same as living within dharma.

Every spiritual tradition has taught that success in life depends upon finding the Way and ignoring the distractions of external things. Your ego, however, insists that your survival depends upon paying *total* attention to the outer world. Its primary tactics—vigilance and defensiveness—are the very antithesis of surrender.

161

*Surrender in relationship is valuable only as surrender to spirit.*

Marriage based on differences can never lead to spiritual surrender. Therefore you need to reframe your perception, training yourself to find the blessing that lurks within conflict. You are blessed when you can find unity with your beloved. The spiritual purpose of differences is to lead you out of separation.

Your ego causes you to believe that separation is necessary. You push your beloved away whenever you make statements such as these:

> I don't care what you think. I don't care what you want.
> This is how I'm going to do it. You can do it your way if
> you want.
> I'm responsible for my own needs. You should be, too.
> If you do that, I'm going to do this.

These may seem like brutal, confrontational statements, but I've simply stripped ordinary ego talk to its bare essentials. Of course we've all learned to be polite about our ego needs, unless we're pressed to the wall. It isn't possible to cover up the way ego creates separation, however, as it asserts "I" over "you."

Being in dharma heals separation by making "us" a reality, not as a unit of two but as unified spirit. You are acting in dharma whenever you allow rather than oppose. Allowing results in statements such as these:

> Is there something you need? How can I help?
> I see what's going on with you. I want you to know it's
> okay.

Go ahead. I'll be here.

I know exactly what you mean.

You're right.

When you come from love, these are not just verbal formulas. Unity makes another person's viewpoint completely clear; you understand someone who is outside yourself. What makes this possible is the realization that your beloved isn't outside yourself—she is only outside your ego, he is only expressing needs that are not the core of himself. At the core you and your beloved are not separate, since needs, likes and dislikes, desires, and lack are all outside the core.

> *Dharma is a vision of spiritual equality. When you perceive*
> *life through this vision, separation ends.*

Following your dharma in the deepest sense means not merely adhering to rules of righteous conduct or obeying the laws set down by society—there is no fixed formula for finding the Way. Being in dharma signifies that you have set a spiritual goal for yourself and are dedicated to reaching it. As relationships today struggle to survive, they need a new reason to justify themselves, which makes this broader meaning of dharma essential.

## SURRENDER AND "THE WAY"

When you first think of the word *surrender,* you probably associate it with defeat. This is a natural association from the ego's viewpoint. In any situation where struggle dominates, no one is acting out of love, and it's inevitable that only one side can win. You only have to remember the last argument you were in to realize that arriving at a place of mutual love was the furthest thing from your mind.

THE PATH *to* LOVE

But there is another meaning to *surrender,* as you can remember from the experience of falling in love. Falling in love allows you to surrender to what you deeply desire, not what someone else is trying to impose. Imagine a trivial incident: your mate asks you to help clean up the house when you are watching TV or reading a book you don't want to break away from. How do you frame this situation?

Ego frames it as "You want me to do something I prefer not to do. I'll decide whether to give in or not." Spirit frames it as "I see that you need me." Notice that the outcome is not what is at stake. Whether or not ego gives in, it is still framing the incident as a conflict. Its main concern is to keep power on its side, therefore it must win the conflict. Winning means either saying no and getting away with it or saying yes and feeling magnanimous. The aim of both outcomes is to avoid defeat.

Spirit has no such ulterior motives. It acknowledges the other person's need, but it neither takes responsibility for that need nor opposes it. In this way the other person is seen as real, because whenever you need something, your need is your reality.

*The only true need anyone has is to be seen as real.*

A lot of the time we are lost in unreal needs. Your mate could be asking you to clean house for dozens of reasons. She may be angry or feel upset that household work is all left to her. She may feel demeaned, ignored, overwhelmed, anxious, compulsive, controlling —or she may just need help cleaning the house. The absence of ulterior motives is what marks spirit. The neediness of an insecure ego doesn't get disguised by other tactics. When you are in spirit you don't feel the urge to manipulate, cajole, seduce, demand, beg, or insist. You simply allow, and in that you make an open space for love to flow.

Does this mean that a "spiritual" person always gets up from TV or a book to clean the house? No. Spirit never acts in a fixed way. In general, to hear that someone you love needs you does result in fulfilling the need. There are certain loving instincts that come naturally when you are in touch with spirit:

> You don't oppose.
> You put feelings over results.
> You want to help. Service gives rise to feelings of joy.
> You put another's wishes on the same plane as your own.

These instincts develop and mature through surrender over the years. But if you go back again to the experience of falling in love, you will see that these aren't learned responses. Love already contains them. Love automatically means release from ego conflict and struggle. A single experience of falling in love isn't a complete release, since struggle inevitably returns, but lovers get at least a glimpse of the Way. Whether they can articulate it or not, this is what they discover:

> It takes no effort to love.
> The state of being has its own innate joy.
> Questions answer themselves if you are aware enough.
> Life is safe.
> Flowing with the current of being is the simplest way to
> live.
> Resistance never really succeeds.
> Controlling the flow of life is impossible.

These are the realizations that bring a person out of struggle. Struggle is born of the ego's isolation; it ends when you can find the Way and surrender to its guiding force.

# THE PATH to LOVE

*Struggle appears to be against others or against yourself, but in reality it is always against dharma. In dharma there is no struggle.*

Since one of man's most prized qualities is his ability to struggle against adversity, a life of nonstruggle falls far outside our current worldview. Yet to come from love obviously cannot be a struggle. How are the two reconciled? The answer lies in free will. Humans can choose to end the struggle and come from love—every day this possibility is precisely what you face in your relationship, for example. Marriage is a testing ground and a mirror. It tests your willingness to believe in love as the solution. It mirrors the beliefs you actually operate under, which are either in love or in non-love. Struggle and surrender are the two poles of free will. Because all of us believe in love some of the time but not all, we are fated to lead our lives in conflict unless we find a way to resolve this dualism. Hence the importance of dharma.

In the case of animals and plants, dharma operates automatically; there is no need for self-doubt and questioning, and no chance of straying from the path. Growth and behavior are both innate. The tiger has no remorse for its predatory nature, no empathy for its prey, no ability to change into a peaceful grazer of grass if it wanted to. If tigers are to evolve into different kinds of creatures, the move must occur to the whole species by increments that take thousands of years.

In modern scientific terminology the unfolding of the genetic code that makes a banyan tree different from a tiger lies at such a deep level within cellular memory that, short of dying, nothing a creature does in the way of behavior can divert its preprogrammed DNA. In spiritual terminology, a creature's dharma is more powerful

166

than any single individual; it upholds life on a set path as long as a species is able to find a fit environment for its survival.

Dharma operates for humans too, but in a way that allows for free will. Each of us grows from a single fertilized egg into a mature person as dictated by our unique genetic code. Our genes put us on a timetable written into our cells. Your first set of baby teeth did not stop coming in because you found their growth painful and cried; puberty was not hastened or delayed by your emotional confusion.

Yet within this pattern set for our species, you have tremendous freedom to act, to think, to feel. You make choices that influence your happiness far beyond your prospects for survival. The fact that we are both determined and free has been a puzzle for many centuries. The Vedas teach that human beings are capable of *personal* evolution, not just the evolution of the species. A person who is motivated by anger, selfishness, distrust, and jealousy always has a choice to evolve and achieve a new level where love, compassion, forgiveness, and truth replace these lower drives. In other words, spirit responds to your vision of it, and the higher your vision, the more you will evolve.

*Choosing your own dharma determines completely how happy, successful, and loving you will be in your lifetime.*

By the standards of our culture, this is a startling statement, for we believe in randomness, accidents, and unforeseeable influences. We do not believe that spirit is constantly responding to our vision. On the path, however, these random elements are a mask. There are no accidents in spirit—everything happening around you is a reflection of your current spiritual state. If your spiritual state is confused, anxious, and doubtful, then there is limited power of dharma operating in your life. You are detached from the natural laws that are meant to uphold each person from birth to death. Without dharma there can be no love, because love is part of dharma's upholding force. A life lived in dharma can partake of love without limits. Dharma is a subtle, flexible, ever-changing guide, always sensitive to the next step that is meant for you and no one else.

The logical question arises, "If there is a universal force that can guide my life, why don't I see or feel it already?" The answer is that spirit is blocked by the ego's vision. If you are living a vision of life derived from your separate, isolated identity—as almost everyone is—then a new vision cannot compete. Love and ego are incompatible. Surrender must begin on the smallest, most intimate scale. It starts with you and someone you love, learning to be together without resistance or fear.

When two people decide to approach life as a path of evolution, their relationship is dharmic. You and your beloved are walking a path never walked in exactly the same way by anyone else who has ever lived. You do not take a breath, think a thought, have a wisp of feeling that existed before, and the intimacy you build together will never be known again. Countless paths exist—as many as there are people in the world—and yet, like an invisible guiding thread, each path must follow the Way of living that leads to spirit.

# LOVING PRACTICE

## Letting Go

In practical terms surrender means letting go. Although you don't realize it, reality isn't a given. Each of us inhabits a separate reality. Your mind maintains your personal version of reality by buttressing it with beliefs, expectations, and interpretations. Your mind blocks the free flow of the life force by saying, "This is how things must and should be." Letting go releases you from this insistent grip, and when you let go, new forms of reality can enter.

You only have to take a ride on a roller coaster to see who gets more enjoyment out of the experience, those who clutch tight with white knuckles and clenched jaws or those who let go and allow themselves to be carried up and down without resistance.

Letting go is a process. You have to know when to apply it, what to let go of, and how to let go. Your mind is not going to show you any of these things; worse still, your ego is going to try to prevent you from making progress, since it believes that you have to hold on in order to survive. Your only ally in letting go is spirit, which sees reality as a whole and therefore has no need to create partial realities based on limitation. Releasing yourself into spirit is the purpose of the following exercises.

The whole path to love could be described as learning to let go, but letting go all at once isn't possible. This is a path of many small steps. At any given moment the steps are basically the same: awareness begins to substitute for reactions. A reaction is automatic; it draws upon fixed beliefs and expectations, images of past pain and pleasure residing in memory, waiting to guide you in future situations. If you were bitten by a big dog as a child, seeing a big dog today will make you draw away. Memory has told you, in a fraction of a second, that your reaction to big dogs should be fear.

Overcoming this or any reaction requires an act of awareness. Awareness doesn't resist the imprint of memory. It goes into it and questions whether you need it now. In the face of a big dog, awareness tells you that you aren't a small child anymore and that not all big dogs bite. Being aware of this, you can ask if you need to hold on to fear. Whether you wind up petting the dog, ignoring it, or withdrawing is now a matter of choice. Reactions result in a closed set of options; awareness results in an open set of options.

> *Every time you are tempted to react in the same old way, ask if you want to be a prisoner of the past or a pioneer of the future. The past is closed and limited; the future is open and free.*

Because the mind holds on with an endless set of expectations, beliefs, and images, you could practice letting go every moment of your life. This is not feasible, yet strong signals will tell you when letting go is appropriate. Knowing when to let go is obvious, once you have awareness.

### When to let go.

The crucial times to let go are when you feel the strongest urge not to. We all hold on tightest when our fear, anger, pride, and distrust take over. Yet these forces have no spiritual validity. At those moments when you are most afraid, angry, stubborn, or mistrustful, you are in the grip of unreality. Your ego is forcing you to react from the past, blinding you to new possibilities here and now.

A mind that is desperately holding on says things like

> I hate this. It has to end.
> I can't stand it anymore. If this keeps up I'll die.
> I can't go on. There's nothing left.
> I have no choice. It has to be my way or else.
> You're all wrong.
> None of you understands me.
> You always treat me this way.
> Why do you always have to do this?

There are infinite variations on these statements, but the underlying feelings are remarkably similar. You feel you can't cope anymore. You feel boxed in. You feel you won't survive. You feel that something bad always happens to you. These feelings give rise to the rigid, contracted state of resistance, disallowing the reality that good things can happen at any time.

*Spirit has a good outcome for any situation, if you can open yourself to it.*

A key word to holding on is *always*. As soon as your mind tells you that something always happens, you are in the grip of a false belief. "Always" is never true; reality isn't a vast, fixed scheme trapping you without choice. At any moment you have the choice to break out of what is really trapping you—your automatic reactions dredged up from the past.

**What to let go of.**

If the right time to let go is when you don't want to, the thing to let go of is the thing you feel you must hold on to. Fear, anger, stubbornness, and distrust portray themselves as your rescuers. Actually these energies only make you more closed off. Tell yourself: Nobody ever solved a situation by panicking; no one ever solved a situation by refusing to hear new answers; no one ever solved a situation by shutting down.

In your calmer moments you know this, but the mind goes on clinging to the unreal out of habit and inertia. Panicky people tend to act that way because it is familiar; the same is true for angry and stubborn people. It is helpful to challenge familiar reactions by stating that you no longer believe in them. Here are a few examples of what I mean:

> Instead of saying, "I have to have my way," say to yourself, "I don't know everything. I can accept an outcome I don't see right now."
>
> Instead of saying, "I can't stand this," say to yourself, "I've survived things like this before."
>
> Instead of saying, "I'm incredibly afraid," say to yourself, "Fear isn't me. Being more afraid doesn't make it any more real." (This technique is also applicable to feelings of overwhelming anger, distrust, rejection, anxiety, and so forth.)
>
> Instead of saying, "You're all wrong, no one understands me," say to yourself, "There's more to this situation than any single person knows."

The general formula here is that whenever you react with "X has to be this way or else," you bring awareness in and say, "X doesn't have to be any way except what it is."

**How to let go.**

In overwhelmingly emotional or difficult situations, no one lets go. You are not superhuman; when anger, fear, doubt, and stubbornness are so powerful that you have no choice but to give in to them, realize that you are having an extreme reaction. Say to yourself, "I'm really holding on, but this experience isn't me. It's just an experience that's going to pass, and when it does I'll let it go." Even in the most extreme situations, you can be *willing* to let go, which is a big step in itself.

Most of the time, though, you are not under extreme duress, and the process of letting go can begin. Since letting go is a deeply personal choice, you are going to have to be your own teacher. The process takes place on every level—physical, mental, and emotional—where energy can be stuck or held, and no two people have exactly the same issues. You may feel comfortable with a lot more physical release than I do; I may feel comfortable with a lot more emotional release than you do. Finding the right personal balance is important.

**Letting go physically.**

Letting go physically is a matter of stress release. Under stress your body tenses and contracts; breathing gets ragged and shallow; hormonal balances switch from their normal levels to the hypervigilant state of fight or flight. You cannot cope with all of this at once. In the overall plan taking part in a stress management program is a long-term commitment you should make, whether through meditation, yoga, or countless other options. Stress is ongoing; therefore reducing stress also needs to be ongoing.

In the short run letting go of stress involves relaxing. Take deep, measured breaths, letting the breath go free on the exhale. Lie down if you can and allow release to take place for as long as it needs to.

Signs of good release are yawning, sighing, silent sobs, coughing, sneezing, and feeling sleepy. Let your body do any or all of these things.

Other means of physical release besides breathing include laughing, screaming, shouting, taking a walk, swimming, taking a long bath, dancing, and doing aerobics. Shaking out the stress does in fact work, at least partially. The intention here is to let your body release what it wants to. Your body doesn't like holding on to stress; it does so essentially at the urging of the mind. Taking your mind off the situation and letting your body release its excess energies is a valuable step.

Under really extreme stress, walk away from the situation—tell anyone else who is involved that you need to be alone for a while to get your bearings. Offer reassurance that you will be back, and even if the other person puts pressure on you to stay, give yourself permission to do what you need to do for your own well-being.

### Letting go mentally.

I have already said a great deal about how the mind holds on through beliefs, expectations, and interpretations. It takes a lifetime to build up these conditioned responses, but dismantling them occurs moment by moment. The present is the right time to begin. When you find yourself in a situation in which you are certain of disaster, loss, hurt, or any other negative outcome, use the following formulas, as appropriate:

> This is just an experience. I'm here on earth to have
> experiences. Nothing is wrong.
> My higher Self knows what is going on. This situation is
> for my benefit, even if I can't see that now.
> My fears may come true, but the outcome will not destroy
> me. It may even be good. I'll wait and see.

I'm having a strong reaction now, but it isn't the real me. It
    will pass.
Whatever I'm afraid of losing is meant to go. I will be
    better off when new energies come in.
Whatever fear says, nothing can destroy me. When people
    fall they don't break, they bounce.
Change is inevitable. Resisting change doesn't work.
There is something here for me, if I have the awareness to
    find it.
The things I fear the most have already happened.
I don't want to hold on anymore. My purpose is to let go
    and welcome what is to come.
Life is on my side.
I am loved; therefore I am safe.

These aren't just formulations, they are new beliefs that, when sincerely held, call in spirit to aid you. To build a new reality you need
new mental structures. The situations that your ego resists with all
its might are precisely the ones that should be embraced, because
from the spiritual perspective anything that dismantles your limiting
mental constructs is beneficial. You have to break down the known
to enable the unknown to enter.

### Letting go emotionally.
Emotions are more stubborn than thoughts. The glue that holds
you fast to your old beliefs and expectations is emotion. Whenever
you tell yourself that you can't let go, you are making an emotional
statement. In reality you can let go of any situation any time. "I
can't" really means, "I fear the emotional consequences if I do." Your
ego draws a line in the sand and insists that you will not survive the
inner feelings that will arise if the line is crossed.

A powerful limitation is being self-imposed here, and at bottom it isn't true. You *will* survive any emotion; indeed, whatever you consider to be too much fear, too much loss, too much humiliation, too much disapproval, too much rejection has already happened. You have crossed the line many times, otherwise you wouldn't know where to draw it. What your ego is really saying is that you can't cross the line *again*. From spirit's point of view, however, you don't have to.

There is a law in the unconscious that whatever you avoid will come back, and the more you avoid it, the stronger its return. People who swear that they will never be that afraid again, that angry, that devastated are only setting themselves up for the return of fear, anger, and devastation. The refusal to face this fact creates much unnecessary misery.

*Instead of resisting any emotion, the best way to dispel it is to enter it fully, embrace it, and see through your resistance.*

Painful emotions don't come back for external reasons. They return because they are part of you; you created them before pushing them away. Every emotion you experience is yours.

We all make the mistake of believing that something "out there" makes us afraid, angry, depressed, anxious, and so on. In truth events "out there" are only triggers. The cause of every emotion is "in here," which means that inner work can heal it.

Deciding to do the inner work is the first and most important step. Even after years of emotional healing, there will be moments when you are certain that someone else is responsible for making you feel a certain way. Dedication to inner work means refusing to accept this perspective ever, no matter how often it returns. Spiritually, you are the creator of your reality. You are the interpreter, the seer, the decision-maker, the chooser. When you find yourself dominated by a negative emotion, try to release it physically first, since bodily effects are half or more of what you're feeling.

Having done that, use the following formulas to reframe your emotion, as they apply:

> *Instead of telling yourself that your emotion is bad, ask it what it has to tell you.* Every emotion exists for a reason, and the reason is always to help you. Emotions are here to serve.
> *Instead of pushing an emotion away, tell it you want to have a closer look.* Ask it to reveal itself from behind its mask. Very often you will find that emotions are layered. Anger masks fear; fear masks hurt. Getting past an emotion means getting through its layers to the root.
> *If a feeling is overwhelming, say to yourself, "I want to ride this out first before I look at it."* Realize that the overwhelming feeling isn't the real you; it's something you're going through.
> *If you recognize that certain situations always bring the same reaction, ask what you need to learn in order for that reaction to change.* Repetition is like a knock on the door—it stops when you open the door and greet what's on the other side.
> *Whenever you find yourself drawing a line in the sand, stop doing it.* Resisting only makes things worse. Let the emotion rise. Release it by crying, screaming, losing your temper, shaking with fear—whatever it takes. Emotions come and go. Realize that each one has a rhythm, and allow yourself to be in that rhythm. The best way not to drown is to ride the wave.

As you begin to master the art of letting go, with patience, dedication, and love, your reality will change. It has no choice.

Things "out there" are always mirrors of what's going on "in here." In the process of letting go you will lose many things from the past, but you will find yourself. It will not be a self made of beliefs, expectations, and interpretations, for these things come and go. It will be a permanent Self, rooted in awareness and creativity. Once you have captured this, you have captured the world.

# In Our Lives

## What About Me?

Della and Frank had gotten to the point where everything seemed to turn into an argument, but at least they agreed on one thing: each of them was married to the most selfish person in the world. They were becoming masters of biting sarcasm and had developed thick enough skins to take what the other dished out. Keeping up appearances in front of other people was still possible with effort, but there were mornings when the only communication between Della and Frank was a terse note left on the breakfast table.

"We're still sleeping in the same bed," Della said. "We have our good days and even some good weeks, but for some reason we can't stop going at each other."

Some of their friends muttered "lawyers" and left it at that. Della had met Frank on the law review staff at the end of law school, eight years ago. Theirs wasn't a smooth road to marriage—it was more like the cautious courtship of two hedgehogs—and neither made apologies for his or her strong personality. They knew what they wanted and never let a grievance rest. When bantering turned to bickering and then started to draw blood, it was hard to assess responsibility on either side.

"No one knows how hard we're trying. Right from the start we thought our marriage had a good chance," Della says. "A lot of issues got worked out in advance. For instance, Frank agreed that I could keep my earnings separate from his. We're very meticulous about keeping accounts so that the expenses are divided fairly. There's nothing worse in my eyes than a woman who wants her own money but makes the man pay for everything."

This was one of the first areas that exposed the rift resulting from the extremely different backgrounds they came from. Della was born into a well-to-do family of lawyers and judges from suburban Rhode Island. Frank grew up in a poor section of Providence, working at his father's jewelry store to put himself through school.

"Our first fight came right after we decided to become engaged," Della says. "I wanted my family to be the first to hear the news, and Frank didn't seem to care one way or the other. So we arranged to leave law school over a long weekend. Everything was packed, and I took out a picture of my parents to show Frank. He freaked and refused to go."

"It wasn't a picture of her parents to me," Frank counters. "I saw the Bentley and the two-story brick mansion in the background. Della's father stood in front like the monarch of all he surveyed. I thought, Maybe she doesn't need another man to take care of her. The one she's got looks pretty awesome."

In Frank's family having a man to provide for you was a natural expectation for a woman. In Della's family there had been several generations of financially independent women. The rift over "your money" and "my money" went deep, despite their carefully thought-out arrangements over bank accounts.

Among all the people who know them, I was one of the saddest to see these cracks develop. There were others: Frank and Della had their own strong opinions about politics, to which they clung vociferously, even combatively. Frank ate meat, Della was a vegetarian. Della wanted to save money to send their two children to Montessori when they were ready for school, Frank thought public schools were good enough. Hadn't they been good enough for him?

"Lawyers" wasn't sufficient to explain what had happened between these two. It seemed to me that despite their raging differences Della and Frank shared the same worldview, epitomized in the complaining phrase "What about me?" They love each other, but love hasn't conquered what I call the return of the ego. Its return hits hard at the root of commitment. Very soon after the honeymoon, if not on it, two people discover that they are not one. Because this eruption in paradise inevitably triggers a clash of wills, most couples have a vivid memory of their first big fight. The immediate cause of the quarrel is insignificant. What is really at stake is the return of the ego.

Complex issues are involved. There is doubt that the other person is "right" for you. This doubt isn't rational most of the time, but reason has a hard time countering fear—especially when it is becoming clear that your beloved cannot always be sensitive to your needs. For women this time stirs doubts that they will be cared for and listened to; for men it often arouses anger over not being supported.

These ego reactions are not completely honest, however. The underlying issues go even deeper: Can I trust you? Will you hurt me for coming close? Why haven't you kept me from feeling lonely and afraid? "You're so inconsiderate" is code for "Why can't you help me?" Della and Frank were stranded at this juncture, which made forward progress in their commitment to each other impossible. We had a chance to discuss their situation when they attended a meditation course last spring.

"There's something I want to suggest," I told them, "but you'll think it's too outrageous."

Being as competitive as they are, Della and Frank pricked up their ears, sensing a challenge. "I propose that each of you takes on a spiritual master, a guru," I said. "Having a wise teacher would provide you with spiritual counsel when disputes arise. You could explore why you're angry and afraid. Most of all, you'd have a source of compassion and trust, someone who accepts you at the deepest level."

Frank's doubts came up immediately. "I don't know, I'm not really that comfortable with the whole master-disciple thing."

"I'm not sure it's right for me either," said Della, "but there's nothing outrageous about what you're suggesting. Who would be our guru?"

"Each other," I said. The atmosphere in the room instantly crackled. My proposal was considered outrageous, just as I'd expected. "It's an option," I pointed out, "and if you think about it, you're both eminently qualified. You love each other, and who knows your weaknesses as well as each other? The possibilities for compassion are endless."

Frank gave a nervous laugh; Della looked away. "I'm not making light of the distress in your present relationship," I said more seriously. "You both feel unappreciated and pin your grievances on each other, which makes it extremely difficult to move psychologically into a freer space. You've become trapped by your reflexive reactions to each other. Your anger has become ritualized, yet stubbornness makes you cling to your self-righteousness even when you're sick of it.

"Now consider, is it really the other person who has forced you to be this way? You've both framed this marriage as a contest, a competition, sometimes a war. I sense a level of mutual enjoyment in this combat, but at the same time it's become totally self-defeating. Winning your little daily battles or even the whole war isn't going to bring you love and acceptance. Mature love can't grow in that kind of framework. It can grow only if you can find a way to frame your marriage differently. Let your spouse be your teacher."

"We want to love each other," Della protested. "I mean, we do, but we don't always know how to show it."

"I don't know how you define love," I replied. "But isn't it synonymous with things like acceptance, appreciation, and allowing? Loving someone means not resisting his or her will, which is one of the first things you could teach each other."

I explained the ancient concept of *Upaguru,* a Sanskrit word that can be translated as "the teacher who is close by." Unlike the guru, who is an enlightened sage, anyone can serve as your upaguru—it is only necessary to realize that each person can offer us, at any given moment, exactly what spirit wants us to learn. When the moment is gone and the insight revealed, the upaguru returns to being friend, spouse, or stranger.

Frank was suspicious. "You're saying I should do whatever she wants, without question? I mean, is this about total obedience?"

"Don't worry, Frank," Della interjected sharply. "You'd have to listen to what somebody says before you could obey it."

I assured them I wasn't talking about obeying another person's will. "A master acts out of love," I pointed out, "but it has a different flavor from the love most of us have experienced. A master doesn't recognize a gap between 'me' and 'you.' Filling in that gap is what he can do, because in reality there is no gap. The distance is just an appearance, all the more destructive when people believe in it as hard as you two do."

Della and Frank are much more complete people than I have portrayed, and what I was saying rang true with their own experience. This was a marriage that had once contained a good deal of awareness and real commitment to learn from each other. Both partners sincerely believed in equality and fairness. Frank had seen his passive mother turn into "the house slave," as he bitterly called her; he had felt unprotected from a father who could be tender one moment and highly confrontational the next. He was therefore very happy to have a strong woman in his life.

Della also had some strong images from her past to work through: two professional, liberal parents had devoted themselves to so many good causes that she had spent many nights at home alone, wondering why she wasn't good enough to deserve their attention. Being paid attention to was extremely important to her now, but she was also aware that intimacy triggered her old emotional wounds. Della and Frank both knew these things about each other; they had begun on a level of honesty that made their marriage much more than a stereotype of legal eagles whose mutual egotism makes it impossible to get along.

In the end they didn't agree to my "outrageous" proposition, but they did promise to keep it in mind. I suggested that before taking the risk of treating each other as their spiritual masters, it would be a good idea to act out their new roles mentally. They wanted me to clarify what I meant.

"Whenever you feel yourself having a reaction of judgment, rejection, or resistance, imagine the opposite," I said. "Instead of seeing an adversary, view your partner as totally on your side. Don't focus on what he or she has done to irritate you; reframe it as an act of pure love, brought into being to teach you the perfect lesson you need to learn at just that moment. This isn't a mind game or a trick: at the level of spirit your beloved acts only from love, holding your highest good at heart."

"Intriguing notion," Frank said guardedly. Della bit her lip, considering the possibility that there might really be a way out.

"Resistance is like a wall holding back the flow of love," I said. "Love is the wave that brings forgiveness, kindness, and trust from the level of spirit. You can't create these things. You can only tune in to them, which is why you need to remake your daily battles into opportunities for spirit. Every sliver of time opens onto the timeless. Can you allow yourself to slip through?

"First and foremost, this is about seeing each other in a new light. I'm not asking you to be at each other's beck and call, or to give up your own needs. Needs don't just go away. On the other hand, projections of blame should go away; there isn't any reason, except in your perception, to make each other feel wrong."

"Sounds good, but what do we do?" asked Della.

"You stop feeding the monster," I said. "This inner being who keeps screaming, 'What about me?' is a kind of monster, a distorted outgrowth of your ego." I had the couple shut their eyes and imagine this monster in detail. It was ugly, covered with reptilian scales, and hard as a stone; it had a horn on its back, which I called the bone of contention. It wore a permanent expression of contempt, and the only word it had managed to learn was "No!" uttered in a loud, menacing voice.

"The name of this beast is resistance," I said. "Now think of a recent situation where you absolutely didn't want to go along with your spouse's will. See this monster coming forward to defend you by putting up a wall of denial, a thousand reasons why you are right and your partner wrong, a ferocious display of withering disapproval. How do you feel when that happens?"

"Hard. Angry. Furious," Frank said.

"Insecure. Empty. Alone," said Della.

I pointed out that both were layers of the same response. On the surface the monster of resistance expresses anger and hardness, but this is only to protect the insecurity and loneliness lurking underneath. If you peel away the layers, you find that resistance is actually born of fear, and fear comes from having been deeply hurt in the past.

"Now ask your monster to unzip its frightening costume and

reveal itself as it really is. What do you see?" I asked. Frank said nothing, shifting uneasily in his chair. After a moment Della answered. "I see a little girl. She hasn't got any clothes on; she looks scared."

"Is she saying anything to you?" I asked.

"I'm not sure," Della faltered.

"Is she holding her arms in any special way?" I prompted.

"She's holding them out to me. She wants to be picked up," Della said softly, her emotion rising.

"She wants you to love her, doesn't she?" I asked. Della nodded.

I turned to Frank. "What about you?"

He hesitated before saying in a husky voice, "I basically see the same thing, but it's harder for me to talk about it."

I asked them to open their eyes. "Once you get past the fearsome exterior, all inner monsters are weak, frightened, and alone. You long ago rejected this part of yourself, therefore it appears to you as a child of your own making that wants to be back with you. Now ask yourself, why did it turn into a monster?"

"A good offense is the best defense," Frank said.

"Exactly. If you feel weak and frightened, the last thing you want is for someone else to see you that way. So you put on a mask. In this case the mask is a word—*no*—that disguises how very much you want to be loved and understood. In disguised form this *no* is saying, 'Love me.' Which is why you both resist each other so ferociously, I think. You aim your offense against the person you really hope will love you."

They were both very quiet by now. The exercise with the inner monster had shown Della and Frank a lot more than they had bargained for. "I don't want you to make peace here and now," I said. "This isn't about wiping years of grievances off the boards with one sweep. But I'd like you to think back to the time before this all started. You are in love, excited to be with each other. The only thing you can think about is the next time you'll be together. Keep yourself in that space and tell me, did you experience resistance back then?"

They shook their heads, neither saying a word.

"Can each of you give me an example of an action that proved to you that the other loved you?" I asked.

Della volunteered first. "We weren't engaged yet, and Frank had taken a long flight home from Europe. He had bought the tickets before meeting me, and by the time of his departure he didn't really want to go. But the tickets cost a lot of money, and he left. We couldn't wait to get back together, and the instant he got off the plane in New York, I was bubbling over with things I wanted to do— go to the theater, eat at 'our' restaurant, things I'd stored up for his return.

"It didn't even occur to me that he was exhausted because he looked so happy to see me again. So we got in a cab and went straight to a matinee I'd really been dying to see. Halfway through, holding his hand in the dark, I heard a raspy, buzzing noise—he was snoring, totally passed out in his seat. And I realized that he'd come out for me, not caring how exhausted he was, not caring about anything else."

"And what did you do?" I asked.

"The instant I could, I dragged him back to our hotel," Della said, smiling. "He fell on the bed with his clothes on and slept for ten hours straight."

"What you've just described is surrender," I said. "Frank set aside his immediate needs because he wanted you to have your desire come true."

"But Della did the same for me when she dragged me back to our hotel," Frank pointed out. "She had been waiting to see that show for months, and the tickets were a lot more expensive than she could afford."

"How did it feel to do those things? Were you put out? Did you hold it against the other person?" I asked. They both shook their heads. "As insignificant as this incident might sound to an outsider," I said, "you were bringing a message to each other that said, 'You are not alone.' These are words from spirit. As long as the impulse of love is there, you'll want to deliver the message. It was there then, and I don't think it's gone away."

"No," Frank said. "But things change."

"Certainly. Being married is very different from courtship," I agreed. "Yet memory has reminded you of some important things here, primarily that giving in to someone you love isn't a defeat. It's a joy, bringing much more to you than you are ever asked to give up."

The atmosphere in the room was no longer charged. Della and Frank had thoughtful looks in their eyes when they left. They promised to reflect on our talk and get back to me when their calendars weren't so jammed. Lawyers. But all of us sensed that the necessary breakthrough had been made.

# 5

# IS ATTACHMENT
# REALLY LOVE?

— 🌿 —

The path to love doesn't end with surrender, although in a way there is nothing more to do. The process of letting go is all that spirit needs in order to enter your life. The rest is a ripening of the union between self and Self. There is, however, still the enormous issue of how two people can surrender to each other completely. No matter how much love you begin to feel within, you must still reflect it to your beloved. Two spiritual people living together don't automatically make a spiritual relationship. Therefore we want to ask in practical terms how love increases between two souls. The ego is not easily defeated in its preoccupation with everything *but* love.

> *Surrender is not achieved until you surrender completely to your beloved. To accomplish this you must relinquish everything that deprives you of love and nurture everything that comes from love.*

One way that people deprive themselves of love is especially confusing because it seems to be a way to increase it: this is attachment. In its mildest form attachment is the desire to be with some-one special. A baby attached to its mother won't accept other women as substitutes; a twelve-year-old girl selects a best friend from the girls she knows. Even in these preadult forms attachment has two sides—it both includes and excludes. Adult relationships carry at-tachment to a deeper level, but the exclusivity remains. The wedding vow to "forsake all others" implies not just fidelity but a life to be shared by two alone.

Isn't it love when you share your world with someone else? Shouldn't intimate relationships be exclusive in just this way? The answer is surprising, for if you look deeper you will see that love and attachment are not the same thing.

> ➤ *Love allows your beloved the freedom to be unlike you.* Attachment asks for conformity to your needs and desires.
> ➤ *Love imposes no demands.* Attachment expresses an overwhelming demand —"Make me feel whole."
> ➤ *Love expands beyond the limits of two people.* Attachment tries to exclude everything but two people.

Most of us would not automatically make these distinctions, because attachment is something we need. But a relationship based upon need is really just expanded ego. Being able to fuse your ego with someone else's brings a sense of security; it justifies being selfish because the selfishness is shared. "We" have our ways of doing things, our likes and dislikes, our sense of being set apart from others. At its most extreme there is a kind of mutual madness—folie à deux—in which two people try to possess each other body and soul. A wild love affair is the closest most people come to this extreme. In ordi-nary relationships attachment seems normal.

The seduction of attachment is that it bestows a sense of security through insulation from the outside world. The pet names no one else hears, the private language and rituals, the attitudes so deeply ingrained that they are never even referred to: these things make people feel safe because they make "we two" a tight, enclosed world.

Yet attachment has a deeper spiritual meaning. It represents an attempt to reach unity by merging with another soul. Although it may not be completely conscious, at some level you realize that you have been living in separation from God, a condition that is full of anxiety and insecurity. There is a part of you that sees itself as fragmented from the whole.

I know a man who was happily married for sixteen years. One morning he noticed a moving van outside his front door. He asked his wife why it was there, and she said, "I'm leaving, and my lawyer says I can take half of everything. Decide now what you want to keep."

This brutal good-bye came as a shock to my friend (in retrospect, he admitted that communication with his wife had been nil for the past few years, so if she had grievances there had been little opportunity for talking about them). He had no choice but to submit to his wife's departure, and in an instant his attachment to her turned to pain, conjuring up sexual jealousy (he suspected that another man was in the picture—wrongly, as it turned out), betrayal, suspicion, and distrust. This pain grows out of the state of separation; it is not created by what another person does to us. In a state of unity, the Self would provide unconditional love, which means that no betrayal or abandonment could harm us. When you are in union no one can really leave you.

But the "normal" state of life, as normal is defined in our culture, is not to be in unity. Even so, it is natural for you to seek to be whole again, to heal separation by fusing yourself with another person— this underlying drive makes relationship extremely powerful.

If attachment worked, people would become whole just by marrying. But this doesn't happen. Marriage can make you *feel* whole. It can bring more security at certain levels. (This is particularly true for men, who often think of themselves as the stronger sex. Sociological studies have shown, however, that widowers fare worse alone than widows, that single female graduate students are more likely to finish their degrees than single male students, and that in general women manage solitude better than men.) Yet the possibilities for unity are not increased. On the contrary, it is very common for two people to feel that marriage has brought them a double burden of cares rather than twice the chance to find freedom.

The question, then, is how to preserve the devotion and faithfulness of marriage without giving in to neediness and attachment. What is required is a state called nonattachment. The word sounds like a synonym for detachment, implying indifference, but nonattachment is actually a state of freedom that preserves and even increases your love for another. Detachment is achieved by not caring; nonattachment is achieved by allowing, which shows tremendous care. Therefore the insights that apply to nonattachment carry us deeper into the spiritual importance of letting go.

> *Attachment is a form of dependency based on ego; love is nonattachment based on spirit.*
>
> *The more nonattached you are, the more you can truly love.*
>
> *Action that does not bind comes directly from love; all other action comes indirectly from the past.*
>
> *Struggling with karma will not free you from its binding influence. Freedom can only be achieved by remembering who you really are.*
>
> *Who you really are is unbounded spirit, beyond the reach of karma.*

## SPIRITUAL ATTACHMENT OR KARMA

The spiritual equivalent of attachment is called bondage. *Bondage* is whatever ties you to the illusion of separation; without it, you would automatically see yourself in unity. The root of bondage is *Karma,* which in Sanskrit simply means "action." Any action in creation—from nature's actions, such as rainfall or the rotation of the earth on its axis, to the highly personal actions of human beings dealing with their complex lives—comes under the heading of karma.

Karma forms an endless chain of cause and effect, action and reaction. You cannot fall in love at first sight—or fall in loathing—without rejoining a karmic dance whose steps began deep in the past. The fact that you cannot remember this past does not wipe out karmic memory. An example will help here: if I fall in love with you and you spurn me, my longing doesn't just go away. I still feel a karmic bond, despite your rejection, and until you respond or I work through my emotion of unrequited love, karma will bind us together. Anyone I love in the future will be filtered through the impression you made upon me; therefore my old karma blocks the entry of any fresh flow of love.

When I am touched by love, karma collected over every stage of my life is influenced simultaneously. The child's longing to be protected, the adolescent's confused longing, the adult's mature desire—all are stirred. The wounds of not being loved in the past reach out to be healed, and the heart's tender hopes flow again.

Karma thus has a double effect: it ties us to old desires and future ones at the same time. This isn't just a theoretical statement. Millions of people struggle with their karma to no avail. A relationship filled with frustration and pain cannot be solved by manipulating your emotions, trying to maintain a show of love on the surface, denying that you feel trapped, or running away. Attachment, born of karma, will follow you no matter how far you go.

Karma has been mistakenly interpreted as fatalism. If you are fatalistic you believe that no action you take will make a difference. Karma implies exactly the opposite. It is a critical part of the theory of karma that "as you sow, so shall you reap." When Christ delivered this teaching, he was stating the version of karma that most people in our culture have heard of. Sowing and reaping are metaphors for cause and effect; the teaching is that whatever you put into the universe, the result will be commensurate. If you give away money, money will return. If you give away love, love will return. The universe, under God's grace, is seen as a place where no debt goes unpaid. Because it stretches over many lifetimes, the karmic balance sheet isn't worked out from day to day. It is perfectly possible in the short term, as we all know, to give away money and get nothing in return, or to deeply love another and be rejected. How, then, is the concept of karma useful in everyday life?

The doctrine of "as you sow, so shall you reap" requires proof that the universe weighs human action and metes out justice. Can this be possible when obviously evil people are rewarded while good often goes unrewarded? I recently read about the death of a Chicago mob boss, the capo of a major Mafia family, who died peacefully in his sleep, having escaped prison despite numerous attempts, over five decades, to bring him to justice. Every prosecution against him had resulted in a hung jury or an acquittal; he had prospered mightily since the days of Al Capone and held sway over gambling, liquor, and prostitution rings well into his eighties while miraculously suffering no harm at the hands of his rivals. Looking at his life, I would be justified in feeling that a very bad person had gotten away with everything. How would the theory of karma justify thinking otherwise? The proof of karma doesn't lie in rewards and punishments handed out by a cosmic judge. When people casually refer to "good karma" or "bad karma," they are confusing karma with reward and punishment, but the working of karma is much more profound.

Spirit would not be love if there was such a thing as good and bad karma, because they apply only to the condition of separation. Spirit is not in separation, and neither is God. The divine never punishes, for what would it be punishing but itself? Nothing else exists. In our perception a Mafia capo is a bad man; in divine perception he is equal with a saint.

Our karma throws us into the roles of saint and sinner, man and woman, king and peasant, but these roles are temporary and shifting. None of them is really us. Spirit uses these roles the way a dramatist uses actors. As convincingly as someone might play Hamlet, we don't believe that he is killed in the fifth act with a poisoned sword. Separating the role from the reality is more difficult with our own roles in life. But the saint is just the sinner in another guise, and the sinner only has to wait to assume the saint's robes. Why do we play these roles? For experience, for growth, to find our way back to God. Ultimately, all karma serves only two purposes: either it is a sign of love from spirit or it is a lesson meant in love.

In the Vedic scriptures the word most often applied to karma is "unfathomable." Only if you understood every action in your life, no matter how minute, could you clear away all karmic debts. This isn't a fatalistic statement; it merely points to the real source of freedom, which is within.

The pleasure of any outward attachment—to money, power, work, or another person—can change to pain without warning. In spiritual terms pleasure and pain are both binding; the potential for any action to bring about suffering is why the ancient sages first wanted to break free from the whole cycle of karma. Lord Krishna in the *Bhagavad-Gita* declares that anyone who lives for the outcome of action is "pitiful," doomed to suffer from the "bonds of birth" and the "fear born of duality." Karma is a wheel, carrying us from goodness to evil, ignorance to understanding, pain to bliss, over and over again.

In our culture, where the theory of karma is not widely accepted even in its Christian version, the existence of spiritual balance is rarely grasped. You have to make a bargain with yourself to believe that mercy, grace, and divine love can be experienced before you will perceive them. For anyone on the spiritual path there is tremendous reward in finding that the promise of eternal joy, peace, knowledge, and creativity is true. The truth isn't revealed all at once, but a day doesn't go by that one's faith that love is a real power isn't reinforced. If you live according to the assumption that there is a Way, the Way will be opened. This is what Christ meant when he said, "Ask, and it shall be given you; . . . knock, and the door shall be opened unto you."

> *Karma can never be simply a system of reward and punishment, since it is the way to love.*

Seen in its most profound depths, the path to love is the same for both saint and sinner, since both must strip away any belief in the roles they are temporarily playing. There is a famous mystical Christian text, *The Cloud of Unknowing*, which dates from the fourteenth century. Its writer, who remains anonymous, says that loving God can never be loving anything you can know or even locate. Love in the spiritual sense involves letting go of all that is known:

> Let go of this everywhere and this something, in exchange for this nowhere and this nothing. Do not worry if your senses cannot understand this nothing,

for this is why I love it the better. . . . Who is it that calls it nothing? Surely it is our outer man and not our inner man. Our inner man calls it All.

This anonymous mystic has touched upon the profound truth that the thinking mind, immersed in "something" and searching "everywhere," cannot reach the divine. God is beyond karma, and therefore so is spirit, since God is nothing but spirit on an all-embracing scale. The "outer man" perceives the world very differently from the "inner man." If I ask, "Who am I?" one sort of answer involves nothing but externals: I am a man, forty-nine years old, born in India, who has practiced medicine in America, who is married with two children, and so on. These are all karmic qualities, the results of specific events or actions that pertain to me. They give me labels that I can identify with.

Yet in some other, more profound way these qualities, even if you added thousands more to the list, do not define me at all. Nothing anyone can attach to me is actually me, not the me defined as inner essence, free will, silent awareness, infinite potential, unbounded spirit. That me, the "inner man," stands outside bondage. It can be "felt rather than seen," says our medieval mystic, and is best described as a "cloud of unknowing." This cloud is like a luminous glow in the heart, out of which a sense of the divine emanates, yet in no way could the five senses capture it or the rational, linear, cause-and-effect mind know it.

## ALLOWING AND CONTROL

If the theory of karma is valid, then nonattachment is the truest expression of love. I realize that this is very abstract. We can, however, restate things in terms of everyday behavior and in the process bring the abstractions down to earth. We all want to be allowed to do what we want; a rebellious impulse rises in our hearts whenever someone tries to control us. These two words, *control* and *allowing,* are synonyms for attachment and nonattachment. If you allow, you let others go in love; if you control, you attach them instead to your own way of doing things, your own beliefs and expectations. The issue at stake is psychologically very immediate, and it figures into almost every relationship one way or another.

When one person is trying to control another in a relationship, he usually doesn't admit what is going on. Instead, his motivations are made to look like love. Isn't it loving to protect your partner, look out for her interests, oversee her wants and desires? For many people this passes as genuine love.

One example is a relationship in which the man insists on keeping all knowledge about finances away from the woman. She is not allowed to see the checkbook; the man's exact income is kept vague; any attempt to earn her own money is rejected or argued out of existence. Although this was a common arrangement in the past, women's self-respect has risen to the point that any man who attempts to impose financial impotence is making his intentions abundantly clear: he wants to control her.

The root of this kind of masculine control appears to be a belief that women are too childish, irrational, or superficial to handle money. (Of course, sociologists have long ago dismissed such beliefs by showing that women, if anything, have a more conservative and sober approach to finances than men. No woman has ever sunk a savings and loan or bankrupted a national treasury.) But this attempt to focus on the woman's shortcomings hides the man's deeper motive, which is his own anxiety that without total financial control he cannot survive. There is almost always another wrinkle, too, that without control of the purse strings he cannot hold a woman's love, for controlling people deeply fear abandonment.

Imagine that such a man is told he has to surrender control by divulging all his financial secrets to his wife, and in addition that she must share in spending his money, taking a portion of it as her own, free and clear, without his approval over what she does with it. This would be the most direct way to confront his anxiety; it would expose the lack of love that his behavior is hiding. But imposing such a change wouldn't actually heal the fear; that can only happen by a shift in consciousness.

Control is the way your ego "solves" the problem of fear. Whenever any of us falls into controlling behavior, one of the following scenarios is at work in the unconscious:

> We are afraid someone will reject us.
> We are afraid of failing.
> We are afraid of being wrong.
> We are afraid of being powerless.
> We are afraid of being destroyed.

None of these fears makes you a bad person, or a weak one. Everyone is faced with similar fears, yet only those people who cannot admit the threats hiding inside cope with them by resorting to control.

A controlling person appears to be free from fear; that is the facade that control presents to the world. We put a high social value on seeming to be in control of our lives, which further promotes the ego's belief that its controlling behavior is working. The unfaced problem here is that control never actually solves the insecurity that underlies it. On the contrary, control increases fear by denying that it exists.

What behaviors am I talking about? In clinical psychology many kinds of behavior are considered controlling—perfectionism, stubborn clinging to a point of view, intolerance, looking after others' needs, being disappointed when expectations are not met, putting up false expectations, possessiveness, greed, and the tendency to get angry if opposed or confronted. This list covers a huge spectrum of behavior that many people would regard as normal. Examine the following list in light of your own behavior:

> Do you keep secrets from your beloved, especially about money?
> Do you dominate conversation and expect your point of view to be acknowledged as right?
> Do you keep a mental list of the times you have been disappointed by someone you love? Do you hold grudges?
> When you make a suggestion, are you offended or put off if it isn't taken? Do you secretly believe you are still right after people ignore you to do what they want?
> Have you generally figured out how things really work? Do you not bother to change your beliefs when you are contradicted or even proven wrong?

In the name of love we all resort to these unloving behaviors at one time or another. We say, "I love you," to someone yet secretly keep a tabulation of his shortcomings. The end of such behavior begins when you see that control is incompatible with love. "I love you" and "I expect you to behave my way" come from two totally separate parts of the psyche—one is of the spirit, the other of the ego.

Protecting someone else appears to be a way of sheltering her inside your power, but at the same time it prevents her from challenging that power or asserting any of her own. If this last point doesn't seem immediately true, think of dictators, who always start out believing that their seizure of power is for the good of the country. The populace then becomes like powerless children living by the benevolent grace of a political father figure. Yet however well disposed to people's welfare, dictators inevitably live in fear. No one is more to be feared than a person whose power you have taken away, even if he or she agrees to it. In order to protect this power, the dictator is forced to impose harsher and harsher controls, putting more people in fear of him, until things escalate beyond control, and the people rebel.

Many relationships proceed on the same basis. In the name of love one person assumes power and the other gives it away. Instead of being drawn closer, however, the couple discover that they feel increasingly distant, for the one with the power becomes guilty or domineering, while the one without power feels resentment and eventually rebels. Control is no solution to the problem of fear.

## How Fear Is Really Solved

False solutions point toward real problems. Most of us go into relationships to find security; we want to be with someone who makes us feel safe. Two people form a better unit of defense against potential hazards and tragedies than one. But being with another person, even on equal footing, doesn't resolve fear. Spiritually the answer to fear is simple: you are already safe. If you felt truly safe, fear wouldn't arise. From the perspective of spirit all fear is a projection from the past, and as long as these projections continue, you will keep generating fearful situations to accommodate them. *Whatever you most fear—abandonment, rejection, failure, loss, humiliation—has already oc-*

*curred to you*. The threats you perceive around you now, or coming at you in the future, are the long shadow being cast by your past.

The reason romantic love makes you feel so safe is not that another person is there to guard you but that *love* is there to guard you. Most people feel that love has such power only in early childhood. As infants we fused love with the presence of a loving father and mother. As long as they were there watching over us, we felt both loved and protected. Once we grew up, however, we learned that our parents had their own frailties and fears, that they were not as totally secure in the world as we thought. This lesson usually came home in a way that brought some shock and disappointment. The day came when your father couldn't keep away a bully because he wasn't there, or when your mother could not take you into her arms to soothe a hurt. Faced with aloneness, the young child is thrown out of love and safety at the same time.

But that is where a mistake crept in, for the one lesson—parents can't always protect you—is true, whereas the other—love can't protect you—is not. Unlearning the second lesson is how you stop having to control other people, for it was in early childhood, almost exactly at the time you were first left to your own devices, that you started feeling the urge to establish control.

Despite its appearance of normality, then, control is based on a mistake, and that mistake is rooted in separation. To be able to relinquish control the mistake has to be corrected. Learning that the world is safe doesn't happen overnight. The world as a whole is far too overwhelming, given all the fear and distrust each of us has inherited. But the love you have for one person is a safe zone and thus a good place to begin. The beloved is like a harbor in which your heart takes refuge. In an indifferent and hostile universe, there is at least one person who understands, sympathizes, and provides for you. Somehow, miraculously, this one person is enough to cancel out the hostile world.

Every day brings many opportunities to replace controlling with allowing. If you can extend allowing to your beloved, the effect is to release you from attachment—both of you are spiritually served by the same act. The key stances in letting go of control are all forms of allowing: acceptance, tolerance, nonresistance. Needing to control life, either yours or anyone else's, is based on spiritual desperation. Look at your interaction with your beloved and honestly confront any fear-based behavior you are exhibiting. When control is ready to loosen its grip, a definite relaxation takes place. The facade of the demanding, critical partner who is so quick to blame begins to melt. You start to feel love once more, not as an idea but as a sensation in your heart. And at last you find it possible to allow.

When this stage is reached with the beloved, the healing process begins to branch out into other aspects of your life. The following changes will often be in evidence:

- You stop measuring people by whether they live up to your expectations. You begin to resist the urge to correct their mistakes and give unwanted advice.
- You lessen your habit of taking care of others without really caring *for* them.
- You become tired of trying to keep track of every detail of your life and bored with people who have always given in to you.
- You begin to listen to objections and disagreements instead of using them to trigger your own opinion.
- Unexpected emotions come to the surface. This usually arouses self-criticism because you can't control your feelings anymore as you once did. At another level, however, this eruption of emotions comes as a great relief.

- ➤ Your impatience begins to lessen. You stop living according to the clock.
- ➤ You take stress seriously, no longer believing that you thrive on it.
- ➤ You begin to listen to your body, which has all along been giving you signals of tightness, fatigue, contraction, and overstimulation.
- ➤ Your mind gives up calculating every move in advance. Some room is made for spontaneity.
- ➤ You stop holding grudges and remembering slights. Resentment begins to be replaced by tolerance.
- ➤ You quit setting external goals for yourself and believing that achieving these goals faster, better, and more tirelessly makes you a good person.

The most loving thing you can do for your beloved, if he or she is dealing with control, is to encourage these shifts, but this is something no one who is still in a state of need can do. In the mind of a needy person, any loss of attachment equals loss of love. In fact, however, exactly the opposite is true. The craving to possess and cling is what smothers love. Attachment is that condition in which your needs overshadow your spirit. So how can you love without need?

Know the difference between ego and spirit. Ego is needy, but spirit is not. It exists to give and not to take. It wants to bring joy; it has no hunger for approval. It does not crave the obedience or agreement of another person and lives beyond all demands. When you see yourself in this way, your relationship will become sacred. Without nonattachment this can't happen. The choice between the mundane and the sacred has always been with us, and it will always be true that to choose the sacred is to choose love.

# LOVING PRACTICE

## Healing Our Inner Needs

All of us bring needs to relationships, but they don't have to turn into attachment. Attachment is created when needs aren't understood and faced. Needs you place on your partner never really get resolved; therefore even if your partner bends over backward to satisfy every need you have, the final outcome will be the same as if none of your needs was met: you will be left to confront *why* you have such needs. This "why" is answered by examining how you feel about being in separation, for the underlying anxiety of separation from God, spirit, and Self is what created need in the first place.

> *When you heal separation, your needs will not reflect fear and insecurity.*

Relationship is meant to heal separation; therefore the proper attitude toward need is that you want to heal. However, in many relationships there is a confusing mismatch between what two people actually consider most important. How can neediness be healed when there is constant jockeying over what two people want? We have to make a distinction between external needs, like food and shelter, and inner needs. Inner needs come down to what makes you feel secure, as tested in this questionnaire.

# THE PATH *to* LOVE

## PART ONE

Look at the following statements—preferably with your beloved—and check the conclusion, right or left, that applies best to you. Answer each item even if both alternatives seem remote or improbable.

1. I would be mortified if my friends found out that I

   *lost all my money.*     or     *had plastic surgery.*

2. I would rather

   *be promoted at work.*     or     *be at my ideal weight.*

3. I'd be a lot better off if I spent more time

   *getting back into shape.*     or     *improving my diet.*

4. I would rather be

   *respected.*     or     *accepted.*

5. I'd keep it a secret if I was

   *looking for a new job.*     or     *planning to have an affair.*

6. I'd like to have my children look back on me as a parent who taught them

   *right from wrong.*     or     *not to hurt others.*

7. In a flood I'd like to be the one who

   *rescued the victims.*     or     *sheltered the homeless.*

8. My problems would be solved if only I had

   *more money.*     or     *more self-understanding.*

9. You're my friend if you

   *back me up.*     or     *listen to me.*

10. If I failed a test at school, it meant that I was

    *not prepared.*      or      *not in the mood.*

11. The worst thing my enemies could say about me is that I'm

    *weak and incompetent.*      or      *selfish and uncaring.*

12. In my nightmare the whole world thinks I'm

    *stupid.*      or      *ugly.*

13. I'd rather be

    *productive.*      or      *happy.*

Now calculate two totals—all your points from the left column and all those from the right. In evaluating your score, we will consider the left-hand column male and the right-hand female.

*If you are a woman* your score from the right-hand column will tend to be more than that from the left-hand. *If you are a man* your score from the left-hand column will tend to be more than that from the right-hand. This difference alone can cause conflict in a relationship. We were all shaped by society to expect security from different sources.

Men tend to find security in power, career, skills, information, intelligence, winning, and physical strength. Women tend to find security in family, a strong mate, sharing, communication, their own emotions, and being loved.

If you have more than five answers from the column that is not your gender, you are likely to be able to define your needs without reference to society's standards. If you have more than eight answers from the right-hand column, your feminine nature is quite strong. Man or woman, you put a great emphasis on your emotions and sense of well-being. Self-understanding is one of your highest values; you put your own fulfillment ahead of external motivations.

Now compare your score with your partner's. There is no right or wrong match here, but your scores say a lot about the dynamic of your relationship. A marriage in which the woman scores high on the male while the man scores high on the female often implies an exchange of social models. The woman is driven by success and the man by emotion. If both partners score high on the same column, they share a similar view of the world, but the balancing half may be lacking. A marriage that is very male or very female can be a happy one, but in times of stress the predominance of one worldview may make it difficult to find the coping skills to pull through. For example, if both partners are so emotional that no family decisions can be made without much drama and little concession to reason, strains will develop.

Finally, if the man is very male (ten or more) and the woman very female, this may indicate a conflict of values and therefore a conflict of needs. A strongly masculine man mated to a strongly feminine woman is held up as a social ideal, but in reality, if the man is motivated by power and status while the woman is motivated by emotions and communication, equality is difficult to sustain in the marriage. You are on two different paths, not a shared path. One way or another the weaker partner will wind up giving in to the stronger, or one of you will repress your true needs in hopes that you will find happiness through sacrifice.

This rarely if ever works. Giving in to another person's needs is actually a form of attachment. Having thrown away your own desires, you will be forced to cling to the other person to bring you satisfaction. This is a form of separation from your true identity, and in the end you cannot hope to use separation of any kind to reach unity.

Now that I have said all this, what can you do? You need to recognize imbalances where they exist and take responsibility for them. A man who has many female needs shouldn't rely on his wife to make all the decisions, while a woman with strong male needs shouldn't ignore her partner's emotions. The object is to find the balance of male and female within you rather than take the easy road, which is to attach yourself to someone else's strengths as a compensation for your weaknesses. We will now examine how this dynamic can change.

## PART TWO

Satisfying inner need has to go deeper than what society or your ego tells you will suffice. To be in separation is by definition to be insecure.

*Inner need must be faced before you can feel secure.*

To be aware of inner need is healthy, to deny inner need is unhealthy. Everyone brings needs to a relationship, and admitting this makes it more honest. Nevertheless, inner need can become so great that it distorts your view of yourself. A person dominated by neediness will tend to have recurring thoughts like these:

> I'm not smart enough.
> I'm not beautiful enough.
> I'm not desirable enough.
> I'm not lovable enough.
> I never do the right thing.
> Something's wrong with me.
> I'm not as good as X.

Whatever is happening to trigger these beliefs, and no matter how convinced you are by them, they are totally false. In the light of spirit you are wholeness and therefore lack for nothing. You are love and therefore must be lovable and desirable. You are unique and therefore cannot be compared with anyone else.

*In the eyes of spirit you are always enough.*

A relationship should constantly reinforce the belief that both partners are enough, that fulfillment lies within by its very nature. "I am" is the primal feeling of existence, and within "I am" there is total peace and security. More often than not, however, relationships are unbalanced. One partner feels much more insecurity, much more inner need. This imbalance is tested in the following questionnaire:

Answering as honestly as you can, which of the following statements apply to you?

In my marriage, I'm the one who

1. Feels more unhappy if left alone at night.
2. Has a harder time making decisions.
3. Asks for help more often.
4. Has more fears about not being loved.
5. Would feel more guilty if I had an affair.
6. Goes along with plans after they are made.
7. Hates to argue.
8. Asks "How are you feeling?" more often.
9. Keeps the family together.
10. Wishes that everybody would come to the dinner table instead of watching TV.
11. Can't help but show how I feel.
12. Writes all the Christmas cards.
13. Tries harder not to hurt other people's feelings.

14. Would rather cooperate than raise disagreements.

15. Would believe a doctor's opinion.

16. Has a harder time standing up for myself.

17. Suffers in silence.

18. Needs a good provider.

19. Wishes everybody would just be nice at Thanksgiving.

20. Won't call a friend on the carpet, no matter what.

21. Has a harder time asking for a raise.

22. Is more willing to do volunteer work.

Give yourself one point for each answer that applies to you. Now tally your score.

**15-22 points.** You have a deep streak of dependency and seek your security through a stronger mate. You would have a hard time agreeing with the statement "I am enough," because you identify with family so much. Claiming power in your relationship frightens you—you equate doing this with losing love. You are also more likely to be a woman than a man.

**8-14 points.** You are comfortable giving away some power in your relationship in order to feel secure. The statement "I am enough" sounds possible to believe but perhaps not that important. Meeting your inner needs on your own isn't something you've consciously set out to do except in a limited way. Two can live more strongly than one is still your motto. Most people fall into this category, although many men would give themselves a lower score than their wives would.

**0-7 points.** Your sense of relationship is based on ego and control. You prefer the notion that you are the strong one in your marriage over the possibility that you are actually the selfish one. To you, "I am enough" means "I get what I want." If, by contrast, you know yourself well enough that this description doesn't fit, you are among the rarest of people: you have taken complete responsibility for your inner needs and have worked to fulfill them without attachment to another person. "I am enough" is a spiritual credo you have learned to live by after years of raising your own consciousness.

## PART THREE

We are now at the level of inner need where the spiritual concept of "I am enough" is truly critical; as long as you dwell on more superficial levels of need, as long as you lean on a stronger person to carry you through, the anxiety of separation is disguised—and that may be what you need for the moment. It takes real spiritual commitment to expose the wounds of separation hidden in the unconscious.

If you look deep enough these wounds show up as black holes in your sense of self. Like black holes in space, which suck energy out of the universe, the psyche's black holes suck out your confidence, your sense of worth, your certainty that you can survive. When you approach just a small one of these holes, you can experience a drastic range of sensations, none of them pleasant. Mild uneasiness and disembodiedness give way to nervousness, dizziness, nausea, vertigo, anxiety, panic, terror, and dread, depending upon how close you come to the black hole. Sometimes there seems to be a hole in your chest or abdomen, or a suffocating pressure, as if all the air was being sucked out of your lungs.

Terrible as these feelings are, they have no spiritual reality; they are conditioned reactions. Stored-up fear magnifies the experience of a black hole because of the effort we all exert to avoid existential anxiety, fears about just being here on earth. Keeping away from a black hole seems like a good tactic, but it isn't the same as healing. If left unhealed a black hole only gets larger until it becomes a gaping wound. The largest wound you can have is the wound of separation, the trauma of losing love, spirit, God. This is the primal black hole; it breaks you off from the source of love, peace, and joy.

Someone who hasn't healed this primal absence will have no energy to cope with life in any but the most basic ways—the black hole will seem to undermine all optimism and meaning; there will be a floating sense of dread that may not be felt directly but that drains the vitality of existence. This is the condition known as despair. Approaching the primal black hole results in feelings of devastation, deprivation, being stripped to the bone, and massive fear of death. The following is a test based on primal fears about survival.

Answering as honestly as you can, how many of the following things do you think could happen to you before you are seventy years old? (If you are already over seventy, how many do you think might still happen to you?)

I might lose my job and be out of work for a year.
I might lose my house.
I might be audited by the IRS.
I might get cancer.
I might be arrested.
I might go bankrupt.
I might lose my family.
I might get a divorce.

I might be fired.

I might be humiliated over an affair or other sexual
misconduct.

I might have a heart attack.

I might be cheated out of a lot of money.

I might be sued.

I might start drinking heavily.

I might not be able to pay my bills.

I might die.

Total your score—16 is maximum. The aim of this test is to find out
if you are prey to survival fears.

*A score of 9 or more* means that you have great anxiety about your
survival. You approach life defensively and are not likely to be the
kind of person who has found a spiritual vision or any strong inner
purpose in life. Because you are so busy avoiding or obsessing about
all the horrible things that might happen to you, you don't have
much time to seek higher fulfillment.

*If your score is 8 or less,* you have a realistic view of life's dangers.
You may or may not be spiritual, you may not even see yourself as a
seeker, but at least you have created enough inner expansiveness that
spirit can contact you. You feel open to the world and interested in
its possibilities. Whereas a person with strong survival fears thinks
that life is dangerous with islands of safety, you think life is safe with
a few islands of danger.

*If you scored 0,* you are denying reality. Either you didn't take the
test seriously or you live in a fantasy of invulnerability. You are likely
to take big risks that end in disaster, although you would be the last
to admit it.

Survival fear is the deepest motivation for attachment. Whenever
you feel that you have to hang on and cling to something in order

to survive, you are perched over a black hole. Although this is a powerful metaphor, many people do not believe that black holes are real. Let's take a specific example: physical appearance is a source of insecurity for almost everyone, men and women alike. Women tend to express this insecurity directly with thoughts such as "I'm not pretty," "I'm too fat," "My breasts are too small," "I'm not young anymore." Men tend to express this insecurity indirectly with thoughts such as "I'm out of shape," "I can't perform the way I used to," "Women don't notice me," "I'm lucky anybody will have me."

These are all negative thoughts that we cling to for one reason only: we are protecting ourselves from even worse thoughts lying underneath. For example, a woman who says, "I hate this dress," could be defending herself from the thought "I'm too fat," which in turn could be protection from "Everyone thinks I'm ugly," which if peeled back would reveal something like "I don't deserve love." Horrible as it would be to live with that thought, it too is a defense that your psyche will cling to if it must, because the next layer down says, "I don't deserve to live," and beneath that "I am nothing." The worst experience you can imagine is to approach a black hole; therefore you paper it over with layer after layer of defenses. None of these defenses is positive, all are negative, some a lot more negative than others. But once you've faced your fears about survival, there is nothing left to cling to—a black hole lies straight ahead.

Fortunately, the terror of a black hole can be disarmed before any crisis or trauma occurs. This is done in a very simple way:

*Black holes are healed by filling them with spirit. Despite their terror, black holes are just lack of love.*

The following statements express a healing attitude toward any extreme fear, or the need it arouses:

I do not lack for anything.

Fear is always wrong—even if bad things happen, they will
   increase my knowledge and strength.

My life is mine to take care of. I can do it.

Spirit is always my ally.

No matter what, I am enough.

How does your beloved fit into this? You can both take the
healing journey based on the safety you first found in love. Falling
in love removes the immediate pain of loss and gives a taste of what
it feels like to be whole and full. Wisdom tells us that this is only
temporary. Love from an external source can never be raised above
the field of change. The only eternal relationship anyone ever has is
with the higher Self. Sometimes in the mad passion of romance you
can feel as if your beloved is inside your heart. This feeling comes
from having a loveless space filled.

The real spiritual work is to fill this lack yourself, which is a kind
of circular process. The mind can be trained into self-love by being
shown, over and over, that the higher Self is a safe haven of love and
protection. The higher Self cannot protect you until you seek its
security; this process begins when you devote time and energy to
self-love. Self-love grows when you refuse to follow the impulses of
anger and fear, trust that the universe is on your side, form your
desires from the heart and watch the higher Self carry them out,
believe that you are enough in and of yourself, heed the tenderness
and sweetness of your love for others, put your attention on positive
energies in every situation, honor your own needs without having
to seek outside approval, and cultivate the peace of inner silence.

When you put these things foremost in your relationships, you
will help your beloved toward self-love instead of expecting love to
be constantly directed at you. Most of us approach things exactly the

wrong way around. As though we were children we first want someone else to make us feel secure by lavishing us with affection and
approval. But you are the source of love, which is full to overflowing.
When you have done your spiritual work, you will fill in the black
holes that keep you from that source. Letting go, although frightening to the ego, is actually entering into the boundless ocean of love.

I am reminded of Walt Whitman, who poured forth his exuberance in rapturous embrace of everything around him yet was equally
the unattached observer who rested at peace with the inner man:

> I exist as I am, that is enough,
> If no other in the world be aware I sit content,
> And if each and all be aware I sit content.

> One world is aware, and by far the largest to me, and that
>   is myself,
> And whether I come to my own today or in ten thousand
>   or ten million years,
> I can cheerfully take it now, or with equal cheerfulness I
>   can wait . . .

> I laugh at what you call dissolution,
> And I know the amplitude of time.

At some point every love story reaches this all-embracing state of
peace within. There is no way to achieve real contentment, real
fulfillment other than through the Self.

# IN OUR LIVES

## Connor's Story

Connor, an older former patient of mine, came to me recently expressing deep distress over what had happened to Mary Patrick, his wife of thirty years. Both immigrants from Ireland, where they had married late in life, Connor and Mary Patrick were seventy but still good looking and vigorous. After a long period of calm and happiness in their lives, their youngest son contracted AIDS and died. The family was grief stricken, but the boy's mother healed her grief by reaching out to others. Mary Patrick became a full-time advocate for AIDS victims. She worked politically on various fronts but spent most of her time offering herself personally, driving AIDS patients to the grocery store, visiting them in the hospital, clearing the way for them to pay their enormous medical bills.

"Your wife sounds like a saint," I told Connor, unembarrassed to use a cliché because nothing less would fit. Connor had a defiant look in his eyes. "You think so? Then why was she diagnosed last week with advanced lung cancer?" he asked bitterly.

I was shocked and told him so, offering to help in any way I could.

"Does your wife smoke?" I asked, expecting that she must, since lung cancer among nonsmokers is extremely rare.

Connor shook his head. "She doesn't smoke or drink. She is the most loving person I've ever met, and *this* has to happen."

I was silent for a moment as various thoughts ran through my mind. The woman in question is seventy, I told myself, an age not inconsistent with cancer. The general medical finding is that tumors are present in almost everyone in old age, even if a malignancy doesn't manifest in declared symptoms or become the cause of death. We have all become used to the fact that diseases strike randomly from a statistical point of view, afflicting the good and wicked alike. But we find it hard to accept this when disease strikes close to home. My reflections seemed like puny rationalizations in the face of Connor's bitterness. We both knew what he was saying: you try to be good and loving, and look what happens to you.

I asked what the prognosis was, and Connor shook his head. "No hope," he said. "It's spread everywhere."

"How is your wife taking all this?" I asked.

Connor's expression became less defiant. "Much better than I am. She's still doing her volunteer work with the most incredible peace of mind, but deep down I know that she's suffering."

"Do you?" I thought. I could have simply agreed with him to show my sympathy, but we had a candid relationship. We both sat for a while, not speaking. It's very common in my experience that one person's tragedy isn't necessarily another's, and that if Mary Patrick was as loving as I knew her to be, she may very well have found the inner peace to see beyond her "dreaded" disease.

"Even saints die," I said quietly, "and they don't all pass away kneeling in prayer." I thought Connor would glare at me again or push this comment away. He didn't, though. He paused, waiting to hear more.

"What I mean is that love isn't defeated by death. Your wife has found something that death cannot touch, with you and with your son, which makes her situation very different from that of someone for whom the prospect of death is terror and ultimate loss. What if death isn't a loss? Since you and I haven't experienced it, we project our own feelings onto it, but there is another approach. You can fortify yourself with love, not as an emotion but as your sense of identity."

Life brings losses of every sort; death is only the most drastic and unanswerable. At some level everyone knows that death is inevitable, but rather than learning the nonattachment brought by love, our response is to cling—to each other, to things, to life itself. How can you cling to life when it is constantly changing? You might just as well try to cling to a river.

When a grieving husband says about the death of his wife, "It was like losing part of myself," the phenomenon is physical, even visceral. To the ego the loss of a beloved feels like a survival threat, despite the obvious fact that your body didn't perish. Another person was so closely identified with you that you extended your identification beyond its boundaries in time and space. Thus grief mimics love. In both instances two are felt as one.

Connor reacted to his wife's crisis with anger, one of the first responses of the ego to any loss. Anger says, "This isn't fair; it's an outrage." The loss seems totally unjust. If I had met him another time, Connor might have reacted with denial instead. Denial says, "This can't be happening." In denial loss is rejected and made unreal. Or Connor might have reacted with fear, which lies deeper than anger or denial. The voice of fear says, "I won't survive."

Although it was his wife who had contracted cancer, Connor could easily have gone through all the now-familiar stages of dying. In the dying process the final stages are acceptance and transcendence. Only when they have been reached does a person stop futilely bargaining with the inevitable.

Unlike the ego's reactions, acceptance is a spiritual state. Acceptance says, "This is reality, and I am at peace with it." The dying describe this as a beautiful stage, which often has no parallel in their lives. The way is opened for releasing all claims on this world and acquiring a higher vision, which is the stage of transcendence. But the dying do not return to us, and therefore we have to find acceptance on our own, before the crisis of death. That is why so many spiritual traditions speak of "dying every day" or "dying unto death"—these are metaphors for nonattachment, the state Christ called being in the world but not of it.

Connor and I didn't talk again for almost a year. When I saw him next his wife had died. Despite an extensive course of radiation, Mary Patrick's condition had deteriorated rapidly. Sometimes a person with lung cancer can be very active up to her or his final days. Connor's wife had continued to visit AIDS patients in the hospital until she was forced to admit herself. She died peacefully with her family around her, having made her farewells and requested that her last hours not be prolonged by life-support machines.

Outwardly Connor seemed to have surmounted the immediate trauma of his grief, but as he recounted these details his voice betrayed much of its former bitterness. It hadn't gotten easier for him to discuss his wife's dying.

"Have you ever thought much about dying?" I asked.

"Never," Connor replied vehemently. "If I had it in my power, I'd refuse to die. The best I can do is get incredibly angry whenever anybody else dies."

"You'd like to be immortal, in other words," I said. Connor nodded. "What if it turns out," I suggested, "that you *are* immortal? What if your wife's death is trying to show you that?"

"You're speaking in paradoxes," Connor said abruptly. "Most people would say that a dying person reminds us of our own fear of death."

"That's one interpretation. But the sight of someone dying isn't just painful or cruel. It's real. And in the real must be a spark of spirit."

"I think dying might be too real," Connor said with conviction.

"By which you mean too overwhelming," I replied. "In my experience, the anticipation of death is always unreal. What do we typically imagine death to be—extinction? falling down an endless hole? going unconscious forever? But these are all projections. Can you imagine the day you won't exist? Can you imagine the day before you existed? Both are essentially the same, aren't they? Therefore couldn't both just be stages of life that we aren't in contact with?"

"I suppose someone with a great deal of faith could believe that," Connor said.

"It's not a matter of faith. If you enter into the process of accepting the real, which means stripping away what is unreal, you could be free from death, here and now. Our worldview assumes that death is an ending when in fact dying is a transition."

"A transition to what?" Connor asked.

"Why not find out now instead of waiting?" I asked. "No amount of anticipation gives us a preview of death. Fear, anger, and denial are all mental ways of pushing away and rejecting. Why don't we go into the fear, the anger, the denial, and find out what lies underneath? Because we have conditioned ourselves to believe that clinging to life is the only way to face death. Actually it is the worst way. It is a response rooted in fear and ignorance, and only when we stop clinging can we hope to find the reality beneath the illusion— presumably what you find out when you die. Reality is always on the move, shifting the known out from under us and bringing the unknown into view. Dying to the known brings knowledge that cannot be acquired any other way. The scriptures have called this 'dying unto death.'"

It is a commonly held tenet of psychology that death is our model of loss, so that any loss—losing money in the stock market, having your house burn down, being fired from your job—creates a deep unconscious terror akin to the terror of death. But in spiritual terms loss isn't reality, it's a concept created in the mind. When the mind applies judgment to change, what gets created is loss. The sun coming up in the morning is the loss of the night. Buying a new car is the loss of money. Falling in love is the loss of solitude. We don't call these things losses because we don't judge against them. The mind has to choose to "make wrong" before the concept of loss can take on meaning.

The law of karma assures us that every debt is accounted for, therefore nothing can ever be lost. When you perceive that something has gone out of sight, you assume it is lost. But in karmic terms this can't be true—all that happens when anything is lost is that its energy has been rearranged. The falling apple disintegrates to provide fertilizer for the new growth of the apple tree. The gazelle killed by the lion returns to life in the cells of its predator. The cycle of life and death, the rhythm of the seasons, the coming and going of species is happening on a karmic scale, shuffling the ingredients of life from one place to another without disturbing the exquisite balance of the whole.

"Do you still have Mary Patrick with you?" I asked Connor.

"Yes, but not the way you might be thinking," he replied. "I know it's very common for the bereaved to feel that the one they've lost is still in the room, watching them, offering reassurance. Mary Patrick isn't there like that for me. She simply isn't gone. Does that make any sense? Am I crazy?"

"No. What you are perceiving is true," I said. "Does this perception come and go?" Connor shook his head. "Do you see your wife's face or hear her voice?"

"That's just it, I don't. Whatever I'm sensing," Connor replied, a look of bafflement on his face, "it's not the woman I married but something else."

I said, "The woman you married is not here, but what you loved in her has no here or there. It just is. Its reality is part of something whole. I think your marriage fostered the kind of love that has this endurance, because you found a way to love beyond personality— that is a very rare achievement."

Connor nodded slowly, taking my words in with recognition and appreciation. "I was taught by the priests in Cork that when we die, our souls go to heaven. Perhaps that is how it is, I don't know. But Mary Patrick hasn't gone, that I do know. I'll spend a long time trying to figure it out. If that's what you mean by 'dying unto death,' then that's what it will take."

# 6

# WHY WE NEED PASSION

Up to this point I have spoken of the cosmic dimension of your self as a Self that lives beyond three-dimensional reality. But we have not yet fully addressed the cosmic dimension of your relationship. What is your marriage in terms of Self and Self, two spirits being joined? Since you lack for nothing in your higher Self, it might seem at first blush that there is no need for your Self and that of your beloved to relate. But in truth the very fact that you can love each other in flesh and blood has its origins in spirit.

*Your marriage is a play of the divine. Two spirits pretend to*
*be separate for the sheer joy of coming together in love.*

The difference between a cosmic love affair and an earthly one is the difference between play and need. Some amount of need enters into every relationship in the material world—survival is too pressing an issue for us to feel that our life is pure play. But in spirit you only play. Your purpose is not to survive but to express every grain of passion that love arouses in you. In Vedic terms only one marriage has ever taken place. It is the union of God as male with God as female. When these two poles meet passion flies between them. But this passion must be playful, since God knows in reality that male and female are One. There was only one divine purpose in dividing into two sexes, and that was the joy of sexual union.

*Sexual union imitates divine creation. What you express through your passion is God's love for God.*

What we need to explore next, then, is how a marriage can deepen in spirit to justify its cosmic purpose. If we could remember what it felt like to fall in love, we wouldn't ask why we need passion. The immediacy of romantic love doesn't raise questions—the experience is all-enveloping.

Passion puts two lovers in a world of their own, as Whitman exalted in one of his most erotically charged poems, "From Pent-up Aching Rivers":

> O you and I! what is it to us what the rest do or think?
> What is all else to us? only that we enjoy each other and
> exhaust each other if it must be so. . . .
> From sex, from the warp and from the woof, . . .
> From the soft sliding of hands over me and thrusting of
> fingers through my hair and beard,
> From the long sustained kiss upon the mouth or bosom,
> From the close pressure that makes me or any man drunk,
> fainting with excess.

This poem brings the immediacy of sexual connection as close as words can. However thrilling words may be, passion itself cannot be captured outside the moment. In this it is like happiness. Anyone who is happy has no reason to doubt what happiness is. But once it has slipped away, even ever so slightly, asking questions about happiness won't bring it back. The mechanism of desire is even more delicate. As soon as erotic passion gets eclipsed by niggling doubts or fears, spontaneity vanishes.

In our culture, because we define passion so exclusively in sexual terms, people find themselves bewildered when sexual interest fades in their relationships. Sometimes a more mellow love ensues, akin to the love between friends, or we may be left with just indifference. Rekindling passion in nonsexual terms isn't something our culture knows much about. Therefore the secret in many marriages, once a decade or more has passed, is that both partners are struggling with ennui. The fading of passion has led to boredom, and neither person knows what to do about it besides dwell in nostalgia. As hard as it is to admit, relationships that begin in passion's raging fire often end in the coldest ashes. Yet relationship should be about uniting yourself with your beloved in a passion for life, not just for sex. Real, lasting passion must come from a deeper level.

The intensity of human sexual desire is a pale reflection of the pent-up longing that sends each of us on the quest for our ultimate lover, the Self. Passion isn't personal, even though another person triggers it; passion is universal. When Rumi declares that "all the particles of the world are in love and looking for lovers," he has conferred passion even on the force of gravity. At the same time he gives back to spirit one of its most important qualities—power.

Without power spirit might be loving and inspiring, but it wouldn't make a difference in the way things turn out; it would be an abstraction far removed from daily events. Of course that is exactly how many people regard spirit, but the soul is endowed with its own unique kind of power, which in Sanskrit is called *Shakti*. In Indian cosmology Shakti is the female principle of creation, the wife of

Shiva, who stands as the male principle. Shiva does not act in the world; he is unmanifest and invisible. Shakti is the visible creation; she is like the mother tending her child, aware of every movement, however minute, in the manifest universe. In our sexual love we reenact the union of these two forces, and whenever we feel loved, we are actually feeling the attention of the cosmic mother, consort, seductress, and lover.

Shakti is portrayed in all these forms and countless more. The tender cosmic mother is Shakti, but so is the fanged destroyer Kali with her necklace of skulls. Many of Shakti's forms are sexual—it is Shiva's passion for Shakti that inspires her to perform her cosmic dance of creation to delight him. The whole universe is thus a gesture of erotic love, and every dancing molecule is moving in longing for an unseen lover. Rumi echoes this notion when he says,

> There is someone who looks after us
> From behind the curtain.
> In truth, we are not here.
> This is our shadow.

The divine love of Shiva and Shakti is the only thing that is real; all else is appearance—the costume of the dancer rather than the dancer herself.

But what is Shakti outside mythology? Shakti has no simple equivalent in English—she includes the infinite energy of the physical universe as well as the spiritual energy our modern physics doesn't yet recognize. Galaxies spin through space propelled by Shakti, but she also carries silent prayers to God's ear. Shakti flows through creation as the evolutionary impulse that keeps order from flying apart into chaos, but her existence is so intimate that no instrument yet devised can detect it.

When the Bible speaks of "the light" emanating from God to create the world, Shakti is being described, though stripped of her gender. But Shakti didn't appear only at the moment of inception. Creation continues as long as the universe exists; it is the spirit's unending expression of love for life.

*Shakti is cosmic passion, and whenever you feel passion for anything you are expressing Shakti through yourself.*

Although most of us consider ourselves fortunate if we can still feel passion about anything as we grow older, feeling passion for your work or politics or even sex is not the same as having a passion for life. It is not just that life is bigger than work, politics, or sex. Shakti is life itself; it is present in every rhythmic pulse of existence. A passion for life implies that you *are* passion; it is in your very being. Therefore the most natural way to be is passionate; the slow ebbing of passion is unnatural.

If you mourn the fading of passion, realize that nothing endures on the surface of life, where change is the only constant. Things come and go, people come and go, and although they once stoked the fires of enthusiasm, eventually the temperature cools. This is particularly true of sexual desire. Erotic attraction is not a permanent state but an opening that allows us temporarily to step outside our ego boundaries and enter into the love affair of Shiva and Shakti. What this means is that sexuality is an opportunity to be in unity, outside the limitations of the ego-dominated self. The opportunity must be taken when offered or else your Shakti—the energy released in sex—will be wasted.

In spiritual terms, Shakti flows in any situation, not just sex, that arouses interest, excitement, and attraction. The greatest waste is to expend passion on needs and drives that are selfish and without spirit. Among these wastes would be material accumulation, greed, love of money and power for their own sake, loveless sexual activity, and obsession. Shakti is the raw ore of life, waiting to be refined and shaped. Insights about passion, therefore, all have to do with sustaining Shakti in yourself and transmuting it in your relationship to love and union:

> *Passion is the energy that love creates with no object other than itself.*

> *The energy born of love is creative—it makes everything it touches new. To see how passionate you are, look around at what you have created.*

> *The source of passion is within yourself. When passion wanes it must be rekindled at its source.*

## PASSION FROM THE ASHES

"What do you expect me to do? I put myself on the line every day for fifteen years, and now I'm an old coffee cup? It's criminal. I'd sue them all if I had the guts." Jarret slumped in his chair, his outburst spent. I was talking with him alone while his wife, Gail, waited outside. For half an hour our talk had been pointless. Jarret's current situation—being fired after a long time with a company he'd helped to found—had made him depressed and listless. He had barely aroused himself above feeble complaining until this sudden outburst —it almost came as a relief.

"I don't expect you to do anything," I said. "You have money; you can get along. What's next?"

Jarret sighed and looked away. Whatever was next, he didn't have the energy for it. "Gail wants to move to Florida, but I'd really feel used up down there." I knew this couple from my former medical practice, and Gail had more or less forced her husband to see me on the pretext that his depression might have some physical cause. In truth she wanted someone who might productively listen to Jarret's endless resentment without being driven as crazy by it as she was.

"Gail doesn't seem like the type who wants to park you in a retirement community," I said. "Not at fifty-three. Perhaps Florida represents a new start to her."

Jarret shrugged. "We used to do stuff with boats down there. We were just kids." I asked what kind of stuff with boats. "Racing. We both grew up around the water, and actually Gail first took an interest in me when I was crewing on a friend's sloop. It's ancient history."

It didn't seem like that to me. "Do you mind if I call Gail in?" I asked. Jarret shrugged, preoccupied with his grievances and annoyed by my refusal to discuss them any further.

When Gail came back in, she looked worried but not drained or in despair—whatever hope lay in the situation, she was it.

"First off, there's nothing physically wrong with your husband," I said, much to her relief. "And there's nothing wrong psychologically either."

Both of them looked surprised, and Jarret protested, "If you think there's nothing wrong with me, try sitting where I am."

"I'd like to," I said. "Not many people get to stand at a crossroads; it's an incredible opportunity. The trouble is that you are framing it in your mind as a loss—the loss of your reason for living. Was your old job your reason for living?"

"That company wouldn't exist without me," Jarret replied, evading the question.

"That describes why you put your heart and soul into it fifteen years ago," I said. "But how did you feel about it lately?"

"He was wasting his time," Gail interjected. Jarret glared at her. Her comment came as no surprise. She had already informed me that what Jarret was good at—bringing innovative ideas into production—no longer counted for much at the computer company he'd helped to build. The company had entered a phase of consolidation in which management skills were far more important than innovation; Jarret had become less than useful, a fact he bitterly resented.

"Your situation has changed, but you don't want to accept the emotions that accompany change," I pointed out. "I'm not telling you to pretend you're not angry, and although it's harder to admit I'm sure you're also hurt. You must feel betrayed by those who should be most grateful to you."

"Damn right," Jarret grumbled.

"But by framing this as a negative situation," I said, "you've missed the beauty in change, which is that it renews passion. That's really what you need." I asked Jarret to imagine what he'd like to do if he had all the money and time he needed. He shook his head. "Nothing," he replied.

"That's resistance talking," I said. "You've invested yourself in negative emotions, and as a result you've missed the source of passion that's as close to you as anything in your life." Jarret looked confused. "Just turn to your right," I said. "There she is."

Now Gail looked confused and embarrassed. "In your certainty that this problem is all about you," I said, "you've shut down the flow of passion inside you, and at the same time you've shut Gail out. You've taken a wonderful opportunity to renew your bargain with life and made it a waste."

Jarret sat back, looking chagrined. "I'm not here to attack you," I said, "but you've been hurting Gail quite a lot without noticing it. What we're here to talk about is how to use your marriage to make your life worth living, from a very deep level. Your motive for throwing yourself into your company once had passion in it, but now I sense that what you miss is externals—power, money, status, respect. At this point, in my opinion, you're not ever going to have that passion again."

The couple looked stunned, and I sensed that Gail wanted to jump in to defend her husband. Instead, she said, "He's just not being used well at his old company. That's why I thought we could build sailboats or start racing again."

"Because you see Jarret from a deeper level than he sees himself," I said, "you see him from the level of love. You want to bring out his passion because passion is vitality—that's what makes a marriage, dedication to being alive. But your vitality is as important as his, and I don't see him doing much to sustain it."

"You're wrong," Gail said. "I never feel more alive than when we do things together."

"Only there hasn't been much time for that, I imagine. You should seriously consider sailing, or whatever it is you can share with mutual joy, as your purpose in life, not as a diversion you make time for if work—or the loss of it—allows. From my perspective, Jarret's being forced into retirement at this young age is the best thing that ever happened to you."

Jarret looked thoughtful. His mood, which had been self-pitying and introverted, had changed. He looked somewhat angry (which at least had brought him to life), but his whole life had been centered on challenge. If he could take my words as a challenge, I knew he would rise to it.

"I know that a lot of fear surrounds you now," I said more gently to him. "But the best way to get through fear is to find a new purpose, otherwise fear will just increase its hold on you. The highest purpose you can have is with your wife. The merging of two energies, male and female, is much greater than what can be expressed

THE PATH to LOVE

just through sex or friendship. There's a spiritual potential here waiting to be fulfilled. Enter into it. Find out what you can gain from
your marriage that goes beyond individual personality and isolated
need."

I turned to Gail. "And the same is true for you. Make your
motto one word—courage. Love and tenderness are not powerless;
patience and tolerance can produce tremendous change. Yet these
energies have to be used not in submissiveness or resignation but in
passion."

A passion for life is a passion for completeness. This means, at
the most primal level, merging the male and female within oneself.
The marriage of Shiva and Shakti is about spiritual potential, nothing
less.

In men this means the advent of tenderness, nurturing, and trust.
Having a woman supply these qualities is not enough. Male attributes
of force and violence have become grotesquely exaggerated in this
world because men leave the feminine energies to women. Aggression and violence will become unnecessary as the shadow energies
they disguise—fear and impotence—come to the surface to be recognized and healed. Being vulnerable will then be seen as a human
quality, not a weakness that makes a man only half a man. Competition based on raging (and insecure) ego will diminish with healing,
and the ability to cooperate will increase.

The worth of women in men's eyes will rise as men stop defining
themselves as the opposite of female. Spiritually, male is the com-
plement of female. Once this is accepted the awakening of male
spirituality can come about, since it takes an infusion of female
energy before our bodies and minds can totally merge with the silent
field of pure awareness. By welcoming Shakti a man can truly be
Shiva.

For women the journey to wholeness is different, because it first entails raising female qualities to full dignity with male. A woman must build up her energies, so long forced into submission by society, whereas a man typically has to diminish the dominance of his. In both instances what is being achieved is balance. No one has ever claimed that the world had too much affection, tenderness, nurturing, intuition, and beauty—all female spiritual qualities—while it is all too obvious that aggression, force, struggle, and competition— exaggerated male qualities—have gone too far.

A woman needs to allow herself however much time it takes to use Shakti energy to accomplish what has been reserved for the male ego. Shakti energy runs in everyone, but women have been given their femaleness to accentuate the difference between Shakti, which is subtle and spiritual, and brute force. This difference can be summarized as follows:

> Shakti understands. Instead of imposing, she
>   communicates.
> Shakti has patience. Instead of forcing an answer, she waits
>   for spirit to produce one.
> Shakti is tender. Instead of ignoring emotions, she uses
>   emotion to tell when someone else is ready to listen
>   and act.
> Shakti is peaceful. No situation ever requires force.
> Shakti is creative. She creates answers where none were
>   seen before.
> Shakti is wise. She considers the whole picture rather than
>   a few parts; she takes the cosmic perspective, which
>   always comes from love.

I saw these very qualities being displayed in the way Gail approached her husband's predicament. She had the ability to sympa-

235

thize, to be patient, to offer emotional support, to allow, and to be tender. These aren't just ways to find a solution—*they are the solution.*

"If you were as kind to yourself as Gail is," I said at the end of our meeting, "if you wanted to understand yourself as much as she does, with as much love and lack of ego, you would have solved your predicament months ago. I hope you'll be able to accept her perspective for the cherished thing it really is."

Jarret nodded, not quite able to say, "I'll try," because he was still too stuck in his old ways to admit he might have been wrong. But I sensed that he knew he was at a crossroads. Leaving defeat and bitterness behind would be his way to open up to the new.

## THE MARRIAGE OF SHIVA AND SHAKTI

Having already touched on the concept of a sacred marriage, now we can expand that concept by looking at the energies of Shiva and Shakti. It is totally inadequate to call Shiva male and Shakti female, since these terms limit God, who cannot be limited. Our minds are limited to seeing masculine and feminine as polar opposites, but Shiva and Shakti have been married since before the dawn of creation. They are a divine whole that chooses to express itself by taking on the appearance of being masculine and feminine.

You and I do the same thing. Although my body may be male, my inner self identifies with spirit as a whole, and therefore my soul must include both Shiva and Shakti:

> Shiva is silence. Shakti is power.
> Shiva is creativity. Shakti is creation.
> Shiva is love. Shakti is loving.

These qualities aren't opposites but complements, which is a perfect description of a sacred marriage. Mature love consists of being able to see yourself in your beloved and your beloved in yourself. To remain stuck in gender stereotypes, to defend one's maleness or femaleness, to aim criticism at the other sex for causing problems— these are all betrayals of marriage's sacred foundation.

*A sacred marriage draws its passion from its inclusiveness. Passion for another person has to fade, but passion for life itself is eternal.*

When the two cosmic energies, Shiva and Shakti, are connected, the flow of passion brings unlimited creative potential. The poles of silence and power set up a tension between them, like the yearning felt between a man and a woman that can only be satisfied by the exchange of love. The current that connects them is the creative force of the universe, which is concentrated nowhere more than in you. You are the ground for this current to flow, it needs no one else. Only when Shiva and Shakti are married in you will you be able to enter a sacred marriage with someone else.

Setting Shiva aside for the moment, since that energy is more abstract than Shakti, let's explore why Shakti is feminine. In our culture a woman's role has long been to serve as helpmate, mother, attendant, and supplicant, not to wield power herself. Power in the Vedic sense, however, is always creative, and creativity is always sexual. Out of a divine sexual act the world was born; therefore the feminine, as birth giver, is the natural vehicle of power.

Shakti can be extremely visceral and physical, as anyone who has ever attended a birth knows. At the moment of delivery the whole room is charged with a vibrant, raw energy that emanates directly from the mother, and the appearance of the baby is like nothing so much as the birth of the world in miniature. Even though the fetus has been gestating in the womb for nine months, this sudden appearance of a fully formed human being is miraculous. That is the conception of Shakti I hold in my mind—the force that can create out of nothing.

Shakti can totally transform, melting away features of our inner landscape and creating new ones in their place. Yogis report tingling energy running up the spine in meditation (its esoteric name is *Kundalini,* one of the thousand names of the divine mother). The presence of this energy gives direct knowledge of God, perception of other worlds, and ecstatic fusion with the divine. But if you aren't a yogi or a mother in the delivery room, what is the experience of Shakti like?

*Shakti is the hidden power that turns matter into life. She is the divine spark, the flow of God's love.*

Anyone who is connected with spirit has Shakti, which manifests in five ways that the God Herself manifests. (For the sake of simplicity I will use the word *God* and apply feminine pronouns whenever I have the goddess Shakti in mind.) As described in the ancient *Shiva Sutras*—"teaching about Shiva"—these are the five powers:

> *Chitta Shakti:* the awareness of God
> *Ananda Shakti:* the bliss of God
> *Icha Shakti:* the desire or intention to unite with God
> *Gyana Shakti:* knowledge of God
> *Kriya Shakti:* action directed toward God

If the voice of God spoke to you, Her powers would be conveyed in simple, universal phrases:

*Chitta Shakti:* "I am."

*Ananda Shakti:* "I am blissful."

*Icha Shakti:* "I will" or "I intend."

*Gyana Shakti:* "I know."

*Kriya Shakti:* "I act."

If a child came to me and asked, "How did God make me?" these five things would be my answer, because this is how God made Herself, or at least made Herself known to us, and at each stage of giving birth a new exclamation of discovery emerged. First She experienced Herself as existence ("I am!"), then creative joy ("I am blissful!"), pulsing desire ("I will!"), cosmic mind ("I know!"), and finally the shaping force that molds all things ("I act!"). Because none of these except "I am" had ever existed before, each came as a revelation.

All of these qualities have universal application. It so happens that the vocabulary comes from the Shiva/Shakti tradition, but any flow of spirit—from lover to lover, from an artist's hand to her canvas, from a musician to his instrument—can express spiritual power. A brown autumn landscape under overcast skies sounds drab, but if painted by Rembrandt it has tremendous Shakti—his kriya, or action, is connected to spirit. Shakespeare's plays are quiet on the page, but in the hands of an Olivier or a Gielgud, the Shakti pouring from the stage is electric.

A sacred marriage would also derive its passion and energy from the five Shaktis, and in the same order as God Herself discovered them. Setting your spiritual priorities straight means preserving being first and action last. *Being* in this case means identifying with spirit; *action* means identifying with career, accomplishment, and the daily give-and-take of life. "I am" comes first because it makes the present moment the most perfect time to be alive. "I am blissful" makes it possible to celebrate life from a joyful heart. "I will" makes cherished desires come true. "I know" allows total trust and self-acceptance, and "I act" makes creativity the purpose of every day.

These five powers form a cascade, spilling like water from unmanifest spirit to the material world. Tagore employed almost the same analogy when he poetically asked, "Where is this fountain that throws out these flowers in such a ceaseless outbreak of ecstasy?" In one beautiful line he states the mystery precisely. What is the origin of the infinite display of nature's abundance? The flowers are outside, but the fountain is inside, in divine essence. To realize this you must become that fountain; you must have the assurance that the flow of life can gush through your being at full force. This state of connection is supreme existence. When you join the cosmic dance, the powers of God as creator-mother fully infuse you.

Now let's look at each of these powers in turn.

### Chitta.

Chitta is God's awareness in its simplest form. When your mind is not occupied with thoughts and emotions, it rests in itself alone. Simple awareness is a divine quality, because in chitta the distractions that disguise spirit are stripped away. In place of complex issues and conflicts, you perceive love as the only reality. You see that you have always been nourished and supported; you no longer need to justify your existence. God's most primal quality is this silence and self-sufficiency, needing nothing else. If we think of creation as a vibrating string anchored at a fixed point, the fixed point is here. Chitta simply is.

### Ananda.

Ananda is considered the first quality of God to manifest in creation out of primordial silence. Her bliss, love, and peace are the subtlest and yet the most powerful of Shakti's creative powers. Grasping this fact is a tremendous spiritual insight. Ananda gives the solution to all suffering, for instead of having to struggle against pain, any person can go within and find a level of awareness that suffering cannot reach. Ananda is the untroubled face of God. When you realize this aspect of spirit in yourself, unconditional love comes as naturally as breathing.

### Icha.

There is a beautiful saying in the Shiva tradition that God created the world out of "His sweet will," which was gifted into Shakti's hands. The Sanskrit word for will is *icha,* which also means "desire" or "intention." Will is the next level to emerge from bliss, because when you are full of joy, anything you intend or desire must be aligned with the divine. At this level there is no question of wrong desires or willful behavior that can harm yourself or anyone else. God can be compared to someone looking in a mirror that surrounds her on all sides, so that everywhere she gazes she sees her own reflection. There is nothing outside this to see, therefore anything God creates is just a modified form of Her own bliss. Icha is like the bow that shoots life outward, giving it a loving purpose and direction.

### Gyana.

Knowledge about God is of two kinds, direct and indirect. Indirectly we can read scriptures, listen to sermons, consult authorities, and from these sources build a reasonable case that God exists. But such a God transmits no love to earth. Therefore nothing substitutes for gyana, which is direct knowledge of the divine. Instead of having thoughts about God, you share God's own thoughts. Her thoughts can only be about Herself. This isn't cosmic self-centeredness, however. It confirms the fact that spiritual knowledge is essential; truth, trust, devotion, and love are inside our thoughts. Gyana is the mind in communion with spirit.

### Kriya.

The last Shakti is the most visible. When God acted She brought the material world into existence. Although both words mean "action," *kriya* is not the same as *karma*. Karma is action born of cause and effect; it is action that reinforces separation. Kriya is action inspired by spirit; it abolishes separation and brings communion. In India a holy person who has entered a trance would be exhibiting a kriya; the inspired words from his mouth, his hand gestures, facial expressions, and even breathing would also be kriyas. Vedic scriptures contain thousands of descriptions detailing exactly which inward state is signified by which kriya (the smile of the Buddha and his uplifted hand with thumb and forefinger touching are just two examples). But in a broader sense the change of behavior exhibited by someone who has realized God, turning from violence to peace, from conflict to serenity, from egoism to altruism, is taking place in the realm of kriya. This is the last cascade of the divine into creation. The stillness of pure awareness cascades into bliss, bliss into will, will into knowledge, and finally knowledge into action. The fivefold nature of Shakti has revealed itself completely.

## THE SILENCE OF SHIVA

If our cultural background makes it hard to see Shakti as feminine, the silence of Shiva—motionless, uncaused, ineffable, nonattached

—hardly seems to us the model of masculine power. Masculine power isn't the same as male behavior, however. The aggressiveness of a warrior doesn't correspond to Shiva, who has no need to intrude, conquer, overcome, acquire, or compete. Although he is called "destroyer of worlds" in the *Bhagavad-Gita,* what is meant is that Shiva absorbs the universe back into himself at the end of creation. This isn't a violent act, any more than it is violent for your brain to reabsorb the neurochemicals that formed your last thought; in both cases the foundation for a new creation, a new thought, has been laid.

Shiva is at least a familiar name in the West, known to be one of the three primal gods of India, along with Brahma and Vishnu. Each was conceived as a particular form of the divine: Brahma is the creator of the universe, Vishnu the maintainer, and Shiva the destroyer. It would be a mistake, though, as I just explained, to think of Shiva as some kind of apocalyptic avenger, or even as a being outside ourselves.

God is within, and the three-part division of the divine is only an image or metaphor for something that cannot be divided. By analogy consider how an image, such as the face of someone you love, arises in your mind. The image is created, maintains itself for an instant, then disappears. We could therefore divide the mind into creator, maintainer, and destroyer, but the actual experience of thinking is continuous and unbroken.

So it is with spirit, which is always experienced as wholeness, but unlike the mind, spirit cannot be assigned a place the way we conveniently assign mind to the brain. God is neither here nor there, inside nor outside. Shiva is best understood as omnipresence, a silent awareness that permeates everything. Of the threefold gods only Shiva is equated with God because God is all-pervading.

In the setup of things Shiva was given Shakti to carry out the process of physical creation. This is strikingly evocative of the way the code of life is packaged in each cell of your body. It exists as DNA, which is silent, inactive, and out of sight, but also as its biochemical twin, RNA, which emerged out of DNA to carry out all the cellular processes that actually build the body at the basic level of enzymes and proteins. Brain physiology is also both silent and active—billions of memories lie stored in the cortex, emerging one at a time as expressed memory. If you expand this to a cosmic scale, you have Shiva, whose creative potential remains infinitely greater than any of its expressions, even when those expressions take the form of galaxies and whole universes.

> *Shiva brings pure consciousness to a sacred marriage. It invisibly makes every action an action of God.*

What would an action of God be exactly? A miraculous intervention, a voice from the mountaintop? Millions of people have waited for such signs and received none. Despite my attempts to bring Shiva out of the realm of abstraction, it would be easy to see him as a ghost, a spiritual concept without flesh and bones. Flesh and bones are demanded by the five senses. When you pay attention to things "out there," you judge their reality by sight, sound, touch, taste, and smell. Yet in spiritual practice there is something called second attention, which attunes you to things your senses cannot grasp.

Second attention makes you aware of spirit. It works through intuition, and it is sometimes called the sight or the gift, although these imply a supernatural faculty. In reality spirit is constantly sending signals to all of us, but because our second attention was never developed, we don't take them in. Intuition is as real as any other faculty, once you have developed it.

What kinds of signals is second attention looking for? Spirit is universal and constant, like gravity, but has no physical constraints. Shiva reserves for himself complete freedom to be what, when, where, and how he wishes. Second attention can detect all five actions that, according to the classic Shiva texts, are characteristic of God when He communicates with the world:

> God creates.
> God destroys.
> God protects and maintains what has been created.
> God covers or conceals His own nature.
> God reveals or uncovers His own nature.

The Indian mind is not linear, and it finds no contradiction in making Shiva the destroyer in one of his forms and the omnipresent creator-maintainer in another. Shiva's five actions are the framework for any spiritual experience you can have; they give it meaning and form. Since meaning is completely personal, no two people have to agree on which action has been manifested at any given moment—this is a private communication between self and Self.

My own convictions in this area go back almost thirty years. When I entered medical school I saw plenty of cadavers but rarely saw anyone die, and I looked ahead to that experience with trepidation.

One of my initiations into death occurred on the public wards of an antiquated New Delhi hospital. I was on rounds, doing the physical workups assigned to second-year med students. It was very late at night, and I had to wake my charge from a sound sleep—there was no other choice, since the workup had to be done before surgery, which was scheduled for 4:00 A.M. My patient was a bewildered villager from the Punjab who endured my poking and prodding with unconcealed anxiety.

"Almost finished," I assured him. I stood up, taking the cold stethoscope from his chest. Instead of pulling his gown back down, the man stared over my shoulder, openmouthed. I whipped around and saw a woman, her face white as chalk, swaying in the doorway. I'm sure the Punjabi villager thought she was a ghoul. The woman tried to speak, but no words emerged, only a sound somewhere between a croak and a gurgle. I barely ran over in time to catch her as she collapsed.

In moments like this a doctor's immediate reaction is to suspect a heart attack. "Crash cart!" I yelled to the night nurse, who had appeared on the scene. She ran back to the phone and called the intensive cardiac unit. In the two minutes it took them to arrive, I held the woman, whose eyes were closed. Then her breathing stopped. In half a minute I began emergency resuscitation with my hands, but that gave me enough time to clearly see she was dying.

Despite my controlled frenzy calling for assistance and stripping away her gown to expose the chest, a calmness came over me—it was impossible to tell if I was witnessing this calmness or it was witnessing me. There was a faint but distinct feeling that something was passing in the air, accompanied by a wave of peace. Before I could think about it, the whole experience was swallowed up by frantic activity as the crash cart appeared. A first-year resident armed with a fibrillator took over, more or less shoving me out of the way.

As I stood up I saw two men hovering over my shoulder, the Punjabi villager and another, older patient I hadn't seen before. "Please, go back to bed. I'm sorry you had to be upset by this," I said. The two men didn't move, nor did they look at all upset. One mumbled to the other in dialect, then the older patient said to me, "Don't worry, it was all right." My Punjabi patient mumbled again, and the other man translated for me: "She was grateful to you."

"For trying to save her?" I managed to say.

"No, no. For holding her in your arms. It made her less afraid to leave." With this the two men turned back into the darkened ward and went to bed.

This incident remains unforgettable to me as an example of the dictum that behind every action is hidden an action of God. My perception of the night's emergency was primitive, but second attention, via my two patients, told me what I needed to hear. Spirit wanted me to know that the peacefulness of death is real.

Now that time has passed, I realize that the message was much deeper: God is present in death. To have this realization, I had to mature in second attention and thereby learn the basic truth about Shiva: hidden within every action is an action of God.

To know God is a process that unfolds over time. It isn't a sudden experience that is finished once and for all. One can never be finished with God; moments of recognition only serve to draw you closer. Hidden in every event of your life is a possible epiphany about love, as it communicates to you from the source. As with Shakti there are some simple verbal formulas to indicate what Shiva's actions are trying to impart:

> *Creation:* God's love is new.
> *Destruction:* God's love is beyond death.
> *Maintenance or protection:* God's love upholds.
> *Concealment:* God's love is beyond form.
> *Revelation:* God's love is in form.

Spirit never stops sending signals of its intent to us in the relative world. If second attention is acute enough, you can be aware of spirit crossing your path, descending upon you, uplifting you, or whispering truth many times a day. These are all silent communications from Shiva, whose nature is silence. Compared with Shakti,

Shiva is further removed from creation as will or action, closer to pure creativity as a potential. But his five actions do touch the world. Silence has a voice, which speaks in something like these five ways.

### Creation.

From my source in love I create situations that teach lessons. These are always lessons about love. Nothing is created outside my spirit but only from within it.

### Destruction.

I destroy the impurities that prevent you from perceiving love. There are no obstacles not created by myself, whatever appearances may say. Because they originate inside me, obstacles are created out of love, and once you find a deeper level of understanding, obstacles melt away.

### Protection.

As long as any situation is needed for a spiritual purpose, I maintain and protect it. Labeling a particular situation good or bad is not relevant to this act—I protect life for its own sake, without judging it.

### Concealment.

I conceal who I am if that is what is needed for growth. If you already knew yourself totally as spirit, there would be no path and no growth. Therefore some things remain hidden at certain times. In my role as concealer I lay out the steps of the path.

### Revelation.

I reveal myself as needed to open up new possibilities. Time and space are constantly unfolding. If they simply unfolded more time and more space, there would be endless repetition of the known. But time and space are only curtains to the drama lying behind them. The drama is the unfolding of spirit, which happens through revelation.

If you listen to the voice speaking these lines, it is remarkable how the "I" can be interpreted as God, spirit, love, or simply your own nature. You are simultaneously in touch with all these levels, although your mind, made insensitive by its conditioning, may not let you see this. Shiva isn't hiding, since there is no place for the One to hide.

*The greatest sign of God's love is that He wants to be known.*

Now we come to our deepest definition of passion: passion is the free flow of awareness from the unmanifest to the manifest. Your existence here on earth makes you the love child of Shiva's passion for Shakti, and hers for him in return. Your life appears to be a tapestry of outward events ranging from birth to death. But all this activity depends entirely upon the invisible flow of awareness working on every level.

*Shiva and Shakti are eternally married because both are composed of awareness. One is awareness resting in silence; the other is awareness flowing out into creation.*

This is what I mean by saying that you are passion itself, for you marry silence and power, the two polarities between which awareness flows. Without the flow of awareness everything in and around you would collapse into a heap of dead matter. When you aspire to enter a sacred marriage with someone you love, you are expressing your own nature and nothing less.

249

The miracle of love is that feeling a grain of love for another person can suddenly reveal the divine. Such a tiny shift of perception is needed to regain infinity. When I stop heeding separation and follow love, my beloved will be mirrored in my being; I will feel exuberance, exaltation, and joy flowing from their silent wellspring. The manifestations of love will multiply because my lover will become sacred to me; that is why love is called holy, because it expresses wholeness.

# LOVING PRACTICE

## Heeding Spirit

If spirit is sending signals to you, how can you heed them? Second attention has much in common with intuition and creativity. It is well known that both are faculties of the human mind. From a spiritual viewpoint you are always a creator. The tiniest situation in your life is not made "out there" but "in here," from the source of reality, which is awareness. People who believe that the material world is causing things to happen are simply unconscious creators —they haven't taken responsibility for being authors of their own lives.

Second attention gives you the ability to take authorship of your life, putting you at the center of the daily process of making the reality you perceive. Since all of us are conditioned to believe that nature operates independently of what we think, wish, dream, and feel, reclaiming authorship of our reality is a gradual process.

> *Signals from spirit all serve the same purpose: to give you back your life as a creator.*

The attitude toward life of someone who functions as a creator is based on these five cardinal beliefs, few of which you have been taught unless you were extremely fortunate:

1. I am an empty vessel. Inspiration fills me every day, but I am not here to hold on to anything that comes to me.
2. I am here to pass energy from one state to another. Hopefully I move it from a lower to a higher state, since my purpose is to direct everything toward spirit.
3. I do not have to control the flow of reality. I bend where spirit bids me.
4. The fullness of spirit, not my ego, provides.
5. If I live from the source of creation, only good can come to me. Everything from spirit comes from love.

Getting to these beliefs and making them work for you is a goal that spirit can help you with. Society in general is not attuned to such a life, which is why all artists and true lovers have had to travel far outside the accepted framework of social beliefs. Society supports struggle, competition, and ego, which means that it supports separation. The worldview of separation is extremely convincing—millions of people spend every day simply trying to cope with survival. But living in separation isn't love; by definition it cannot bring you to unity.

*Spirit is your chief and only ally in your quest for unity. The tactics of non-love will never get you to love.*

In the following exercise you will learn how to transmute the beliefs and behaviors of separation into those of love, using the signals that spirit is always sending.

# Why We Need Passion

## PART ONE

The voice of spirit is constantly competing with other voices inside you, and the outcome of your life depends on which voice you follow. Since inner voices are constant, you can estimate what a person expects from life by looking at his or her inner voices for a period no longer than forty-eight hours.

Read the following statements and check those that have applied to you *over the past two days:*

1. I was afraid something wasn't going to work out for me.
2. I resolved a situation by acting nicer than I really felt.
3. I couldn't figure out how I felt about something.
4. I had doubts about how someone close to me actually feels about me.
5. I didn't tell the truth when I should have.
6. Someone hurt my feelings, but I let it pass.
7. I had worries when I went to bed, *or* I had a bad dream, *or* I had insomnia.
8. Someone let me down.
9. I thought about how good things used to be and wished I could go back.
10. I felt frustrated by some part of my life that's gotten out of control.
11. I regretted something I said.
12. I felt bad about my feelings.
13. I talked behind someone's back.
14. I complained to someone who couldn't help the situation I was in.
15. Someone bothered me, but I didn't confront them.
16. I was afraid to ask for what I wanted.
17. I didn't say, "I love you."
18. I felt bad about myself.

19. I looked at the news on TV and thought things were really getting worse.
20. Nothing seemed to go right.

Each check counts as a point. Total your score, which will fall into one of these three broad categories:

**0 – 5 points.** You live in the present and do not heed strong inner voices of fear or guilt. Your self-worth is based upon real expectations. You are not stuck reliving past emotions or trying to atone for past mistakes. Others may marvel at how low your stress is, but you work to keep it that way every day.

**6 – 15 points.** You tend to listen to inner voices that are not you but are expressions of your fear, anger, and disappointment. You have a habit of not being totally truthful about your emotions, either to yourself or to others. Self-doubt is a problem that increases for you as your stress mounts. If there's a choice between what you want to do and what you think you'd better do in order to be safe or to go along with others, you'll take the second choice. In times of conflict or crisis, you will escape by watching TV or complaining to friends rather than sit and work out what you can do to change the situation. You say things like "It'll all work out" when deep inside you are quite afraid that it won't.

**16 – 20 points.** You have a hard time telling where your inner voices leave off and you begin. You hate confrontation because it means actually being honest with yourself or other people. Getting along is very important to you. You find yourself saying things you don't mean; you make promises you regret afterward. Sometimes you look around and wonder what kinds of friends you have and feel that you don't really know them—which means that you do not get close to people or allow them to get close to you. Blaming your parents comes all too easily, or you want to run back to them when things get rough. Your core beliefs have yet to surface, but if they did, you would believe that survival is a dangerous business and love has little force in this world.

The whole business of inner voices is highly complex, but from spirit's viewpoint the only inner voice you need to follow is that of the higher Self. To see if you are heeding that voice, read the next list of statements and check which ones have applied to you *over the last two days:*

1. I decided to go it alone on something that matters to me.
2. I had a great new idea.
3. I came up with a way to solve a situation out of nowhere.
4. I said, "I love you."
5. I got something off my chest I'd wanted to say for a while.
6. I swallowed my pride and admitted I was wrong.
7. I supported someone who was in doubt or wanted to make a difficult change.
8. I stood up for myself, even though I felt nervous about it.
9. Despite the evening news I feel that life is good.
10. I didn't blame anyone.
11. I didn't complain.
12. I searched deep inside.
13. I made someone feel better about themselves than they did before.
14. I saw something good in someone who had made a bad impression on me before.

15. I trusted and it worked out.
16. My faith in God was justified.
17. I had a moment of insight.
18. I forgave myself, *or* I was kind to myself.
19. I was tempted to jump to conclusions but didn't.
20. I was at peace.

Give yourself a point for each statement you checked and total your score.

**0-5 points.** Your life is based on values other than spiritual. You may be unaware of this because you have success, money, and a good family life—or you may not be unaware. In either case your inner climate is dominated by routine. Creativity and sensitivity are not high on the list of things you value, or you don't see yourself being creative. Looking deep inside isn't something you do very often, since you are afraid of what you might find. "Love" to you means having your needs fulfilled by another person. You are likely to describe yourself as an atheist, pessimist, or skeptic.

**6-15 points.** You attend church or at least believe in God, but you do not have a strong personal link to spirit. You are not driven by success or money, which gives you some peace of mind, but you haven't found a real passion at the core of yourself. Problems don't overwhelm you if they aren't too big, but you don't expect to come up with major innovations or creative accomplishments either. Being on safe middle ground is all right with you, although you sometimes fear for the future. "Love" to you means a secure family, a devoted spouse, and feeling good about people.

**16-20 points.** You are in tune with spirit. Conventional religious beliefs matter much less to you than active participation in your own creative lifestyle. Your belief in God is founded on experience, but at the same time you consider yourself the author of your own existence. In a crisis you may be shaken, but when the emotions clear you look for positive outcomes and almost always find them. You think in terms not of being safe but of what you want to do and want to be—you follow your star. "Love" to you means a force beyond personality that can be seen and felt everywhere you look, if only you look hard enough.

In most cases scoring high on either of these tests means that you scored low on the other, because following the voice of spirit is the opposite of following the voices of fear, anger, and doubt. Spirit's voice is harder to follow because it is neither loud nor demanding, whereas the voice of fear, for instance, is extremely loud and at times overwhelming in its insistence. Other voices are from the past: your thoughts are not really your own but borrowed from authority figures who once had influence over you. These voices say, "This is what you'd better do"—they warn and often punish. Other voices from the past express habits and beliefs. When someone exclaims, "If I listen to myself, I hear my mother talking," what he really means is that an adopted belief system is having its say; the source of these beliefs—father, mother, coach, teacher, guru—still has a voice in your head, repeating the tenets you are holding on to.

But it is you who holds on. You are the one who decides which voice to heed, which to reject. A vast majority of the time, people do not heed the voice that makes them either happy or loving. They are led into unloving and unhappy outcomes because they followed the wrong voice, and they spend immense amounts of time in therapy basically to get these wrong voices out of their heads.

The next exercise will help you to recognize when spirit is speaking to you and how to heed it.

## PART TWO

Getting rid of the negative voices in your head isn't accomplished by arguing with them, ignoring them, or trying to pretend that they aren't there. It involves a process of letting go; the Loving Practice "Letting Go" (p. 169) details how this process works. Here I will be concerned with how to attune yourself to the voice of spirit. Spirit is hard to listen to if you are enmeshed in your old beliefs and social conditioning, for the following reasons:

- Spirit is not verbal like the other thoughts in your head. It comes as insight, an "aha!" that makes you see things in a new light.
- Spirit doesn't argue or try to persuade. It shows you what is real in a given situation, pure and simple.
- Spirit doesn't say, "If you don't do this, that will follow." There are no ultimatums or threats.
- Spirit doesn't communicate in terms of right and wrong. Whatever you decide to do, spirit will support you.
- Spirit always makes you feel better about yourself, but it may pose choices that take courage, patience, and faith.
- You can't make spirit do anything. It speaks when it wants to, but you can be sure that it will speak at the right time.
- Spirit never comes from anything but love. If you are looking for a way to find revenge, to prove yourself right, to oppose or conquer others, or to punish, the voice in your head isn't spirit.

These are the guidelines that enable you to tune in to your second attention. First attention is dominated by outside events, by expectations about the way things should turn out, and by old conditioning—if you detect any of these influences, you know you aren't in spirit. Ask yourself the following questions any time you have a doubt about this:

> Am I angry or anxious?
>
> Am I suspicious or doubtful?
>
> Do I feel overwhelmed by what's going on around me?
>
> Is somebody else trying to make up my mind
>     for me?
>
> Is my body tense or feeling discomfort?
>
> Has this happened to me before? Am I just repeating a past
>     scenario?
>
> Do I have to have things turn out a certain way?
>
> Do I feel I'm in danger?

These are signals from your ego, far removed from spirit despite the fact that we act on such signals all the time. It is in the *absence* of these ego signals that spirit is speaking to you. One kind of signal can't be converted to the other. Transmuting your behavior from ego based to spirit based means cultivating your second attention. If you act on spirit you will see results that you never expected, such as these:

> Your fears will no longer come true.
>
> Your happiness will no longer depend on expectations.
>
> You will feel safe.
>
> You will feel loved.

As you begin to heed spirit, you can only increase in love—passion for life will appear naturally. We are like empty vessels being endlessly refilled with spirit. To be in love with someone is to share this inexhaustible flow. Love shares awareness and being; it is a silent communication that unites two people more and more in a spiritual reality unknown outside their intimacy. They have reclaimed their lives by becoming authors of their own reality.

# IN OUR LIVES

## Wooing the Goddess

"I'm sure you don't want to hear my problems," Amy began. "Another boring, weepy wife. How many have you met as a doctor—a hundred? A thousand?" She sounded distraught.

"Is boring how you feel?" I asked. Amy's eyes turned dull.

"It doesn't matter much how I feel," she said. After twenty years of marriage to a CEO from San Diego named Fred, Amy considered herself a discarded wife.

"Is Fred seeing someone else? Does he want a divorce?" I asked. Amy shook her head.

"I don't know what he wants. We don't see each other much these days. I'm alone until he is driven home after six, if he can make it home at all. He might as well have a cellular phone grafted to his ear for all he pays attention when he is around. And going to bed means going to sleep."

"Do you think Fred wants this situation to change?" I asked.

"Why should he? His life's exciting. I'm a boring holdover from his past." Amy looked sad, but instead of crying she sighed and squared her shoulders.

"You've used the word *boring* twice," I pointed out. "Is that something we could talk about?"

Amy shrugged and looked away. "I guess," she said.

"Since we all tend to find it easier to look outward than inward," I said, "we rarely challenge the notion that there are 'boring' people and 'boring' situations. When someone complains that her or his marriage has become boring, the usual remedy is external. The woman decides she needs to look more seductive, so she buys a flimsy negligee, turns down the lights, and puts on mood music. The man brings home candy and flowers and vows to take his wife dancing."

A half smile crossed Amy's face, as if to say, "We're way beyond that."

I went on. "Being external, these can be only superficial gestures. The heart of the problem is not a boring relationship (and by implication, a boring partner), but a failure to discover where passion comes from and how it is kept alive. What you're talking about here is the fading of passion. Is it really all on Fred's side? How exciting is he?"

"That doesn't seem to matter," Amy said. "Not to him."

"You just feel guiltier than he does," I said. "I'd be surprised if he felt any more desirable than you do right now."

Amy looked surprised; it was clear that she was resigned to a boring marriage and that she had taken all the blame for that upon herself.

"Before asking the question 'Where did the passion go?'" I said, "you first have to ask, 'Why did I want it to go?' Passion is the flow of life, in all its natural exuberance. Passion doesn't just fade; it gets blocked, and you have to ask why you blocked it." I didn't wait for Amy to answer, since she looked baffled. "The answer, almost always, is rooted in the past. To a surprising extent we have all learned to approach passion with caution, as something that may hurt us. An unconscious censor inside your mind decides whether it is permissible for you to feel passionate or not."

"I've always suspected that Fred thinks I'm cold," Amy said. "We used to disagree a lot about how much sex is 'normal.' "

"Meaning that you got tagged as wanting too little?" I asked. Her silence was answer enough. "This issue of how much sex is too little or too much is a diversionary tactic," I said. "Normal is however much two people feel comfortable with, as long as there is love. Could the real issue be that sex wasn't so good for you, so you gradually wanted less of it?"

"Fred's not the champion he thinks he is," Amy said with sudden resentment. She stopped herself, biting her lip.

"Fred's very competitive," I pointed out, "and performance is extremely important to such men. Tenderness doesn't come easily to them, nor does sensitivity to their partners. But the blame can always be shifted by claiming that the woman is undersexed or that the man has too much libido. Again the real issue isn't too much or too little. It's how much emotion you feel safe expressing through sexual activity—in other words, how much you judge against passion."

"I don't judge against it," Amy protested.

"You judge against your emotions, which amounts to the same thing," I said.

*Sex is always about emotions. Good sex is about free emotions; bad sex is about blocked emotions.*

"So what is it that blocks the flow of emotion? This blockage is felt as boredom, which is what both you and Fred feel."

"Maybe I am just boring," Amy said.

"No, that is guilt, which is holding back a lot of anger," I said. "Boredom is never a primary feeling; it arises from a much more basic response, an inner hurt that has disconnected you from yourself.

THE PATH *to* LOVE

Boredom begins when you allow yourself to feel little or no emotional stimulation, and from there stem the reactions of dullness, lethargy, and depression.

"Listen," I said. "Everything you want from Fred you can give yourself." Amy looked at me with disbelief. "Pinning your frustrations on your mate is like pinning your happiness on him, only in reverse, and neither will work. Where are you going to find passion if not in yourself? Having found it, you can give to Fred in the way you want him to give to you. That is always the solution."

I suggested that we leave Fred entirely out of it for the moment and talk more about emotions. "How do you feel about yourself right now?" I asked.

"I'm afraid to tell you," Amy said with a twisted smile.

"Because you're going to say 'boring,' right?" She nodded. "Boredom is a kind of numbness," I pointed out. "A person who says, 'I have no feelings' really means, 'I can't find my feelings anymore.' "

Clearly I had struck a chord. Amy began to tell me of nights when she was afraid she felt nothing for Fred, when their lovemaking was so perfunctory that she couldn't wait for it to be over.

"But what was the feeling you were pushing aside?" I asked. "If you look deep enough you'll find that it was hurt. That would be the most natural feeling for anyone—man or woman—whose partner isn't really making love. Love is not about orgasm; it's about surrender to the other person, and Fred doesn't sound like he was ever capable of surrender."

"I'm not sure he knows the concept," Amy said softly. Clearly no one had told Fred that noticing someone else's emotions is the essence of communication. But it struck me that Amy's feelings, or lack of them, had to be addressed first.

"Let's try to understand something," I suggested. "Why do you feel one way and somebody else another? We have to go back to this whole question of boundaries. In most cases early childhood taught us that being cold and self-contained was preferable to being emotional. Passion came to be equated with emotions that were 'too much' for your own good. Children are taught to respect the emotional boundaries imposed by parents. This teaching usually isn't direct, but it doesn't have to be. Without being handed a textbook, a young child quickly learns to recognize when she is crying 'too much,' laughing 'too hard,' or being 'too noisy.' "

Yet by nature all emotion is spontaneous, which means that an emotion like crying or laughing will run its course if allowed to. There is no such thing as crying too much—we simply cry until we are through, and we are through when the underlying energy of hurt has spent itself. Likewise there is no such thing as laughing too hard or getting too angry or grieving beyond measure.

The limits we impose on all our emotions originated with the discomfort of our parents. We formed our boundaries by reacting to theirs. They also were taught as children to recognize when an emotion was "too much." Their sense of appropriateness was inherited, and they had little choice but to pass it on.

"What this means," I told Amy, "is that your emotional life isn't completely yours. It comes to you secondhand and even thirdhand. Every tear you shed, every angry outburst, every peal of laughter reflects the emotional comfort range of parents and grandparents, *people who are not yourself.*"

My sudden emphasis startled Amy. She reflected for a moment. "So what am I supposed to do—go wild, lose myself? I'm too old for those games."

"I'm not saying that all emotional displays are appropriate no matter how extreme. If we had been allowed to discover our emotions without outside inhibition, they would not run to extremes; nature respects its own limits."

A medical parallel can be made to blood pressure. When the body needs to call upon it the vascular system contracts and dilates, resulting in very high blood pressure when you are excited or exercising heavily, for example, and lower blood pressure for periods of relaxation or creativity. These are extreme variations from "normal" blood pressure, yet they are entirely natural. The body knows how to accommodate its needs regardless of what we arbitrarily deem normal. Nature's definition of *normal* is whatever your system needs at any given moment in order to remain in balance.

Emotions are released to restore balance in the psyche, and if left to its natural mechanisms the psyche has no difficulty determining when it is appropriate to laugh, cry, burst out in anger, or tremble with fear. The connection with passion is this: passion is just the free flow of natural emotional energy.

"What this would all suggest," I said, "is that emotional therapy is in order here. But what if Fred doesn't think there's a problem? What if he finds it too threatening to explore emotions? Instead of depending on him, let's look at passion from a spiritual viewpoint, with the aim of seeing if you can regain your passion. Ultimately, isn't that the problem? Fred's response is merely a reflection of what is going on inside you spiritually."

Hesitantly Amy agreed to go in this direction. It was clear that long-standing emotional difficulties in her marriage weren't going to be solved by having a talk with me, but the spiritual issues ran much deeper than emotion.

"If we could peel away the level of negative feelings inside you," I said, "we would expose a deeper core. What is this core made of? There are many related factors—beliefs that separation has to occur, habits of being isolated, old defeatism that prevents you from trying to reconnect. But if we look at all these levels, a surprisingly simple diagnosis emerges."

*We feel bored when we can't admit that we have desires.*

"Unless desires are allowed to run their course," I said, "existence feels futile. Your mate didn't inflict this condition on you; it is your own creation. Futility is a depressed condition that signifies, 'What I want doesn't matter.' This in turn is tied to similar beliefs, such as 'What I feel doesn't make a difference' and 'What I say doesn't get heard.' The common thread linking all these versions is that *you are powerless.* Someone with no power feels that desire is hopeless, since it will never be fulfilled; therefore why bother to have desires in the first place?"

Amy is an intelligent woman, and the fact that she had subordinated her power to Fred was not lost on her. As is true of most depressed people she had no Shakti of her own. The five powers all of us should take strength from were greatly diminished in her.

> Instead of "I am" she felt, "Do I deserve to be here?"
> Instead of "I am blissful" she felt, "I can't feel."
> Instead of "I will" she felt, "I can't."
> Instead of "I know" she felt, "I doubt."
> Instead of "I act" she felt, "I don't know what to do."

Where did her Shakti go? The roots of powerlessness run deep. Some people feel that they were stripped of power by their parents, by destiny, by God. In actual fact we all disempower ourselves. It is impossible to exist without desires, which Shakti uses to guide us from one fulfillment to another. If desire is denied, however, Shakti is rendered useless. It takes an active effort to make desire seem to go away.

*Passion doesn't fade. It must be suppressed.*

Boredom is just the passive face of this effort to keep desire out of sight, the indifferent mask put on to hide a huge internal struggle. The belief that you won't ever get what you want implies enormous hatred and judgment against yourself. Keeping these feelings in control takes work, for even if you sincerely believe that you do not deserve to have desires, the vitality of life isn't going to be completely halted.

People who have cut themselves off from passion have switched their allegiance to something else almost as strong. Because the flow of life won't be stopped, a counterforce must be called in to oppose it—the counterforce of fear. Fear of life is extremely common whenever someone complains of ennui.

Fear at any level of the psyche makes it much more difficult to trust that passion is safe. If my wife criticizes me, a warning voice that I hardly notice will sap my desire for her. If my husband dislikes the way I keep house, I will feel inhibition about fully expressing my sexual needs. Thus existential issues are activated by everyday obstacles.

In relationships where two people have allowed the underground war between fear and desire to go on too long, suppressing passion becomes an actual life goal. In fear's warped value system, getting "too close" seems like a problem instead of the solution. As nature created us it is normal to seek pleasure; a fearful person avoids pain instead.

"Whether you can admit it to yourself or not," I told Amy, "being bored is your goal in life. Boredom isn't happening to you;

you are using it in the pursuit of safety and security. Why don't you tell Fred off or throw a vase at him or break down and cry?" Amy looked stunned.

"I just wouldn't," she muttered, her face strained by unwept tears.

I said more gently, "Bringing light to this dark dilemma is going to make things better. Right now your stance toward the river of life is to stand on the banks and try not to fall in. But can you survive without falling in?

"The spiritual answer to boredom is to open yourself to the very thing you have feared—the constant flow of desire that wants to express itself at every moment."

*We are enticed back into passion when we admit to having desires.*

The reason that falling in love is so passionate is simple: desire is no longer a choice. Romance bursts the dam of inhibition. Its erotic power proves too much for fear and repression to hold back. At the deepest level people never fall in love accidentally. They simply grow tired of living without passion, and having made this unconscious decision they open up once more and allow themselves to receive love.

Without waiting to fall in love, you can rekindle passion by imitating this process. When the passion is gone from a relationship, both partners must be honest in stating that they have desires. This of course can be difficult, for if either partner is operating under the belief "I'm bored with you," it will be doubly difficult to say, "I desire you." The critical step is to eliminate your partner entirely as the cause of the problem and take responsibility for your own feelings.

The essential issue is not "I am bored with you" but "I am bored." By taking blame out of the equation, you also remove threat. This is extremely important, because you cannot help but fear anyone whom you are mentally attacking.

"Your whole effort needs to be directed toward finding out what you really want and then feeling you deserve to fulfill those desires," I told Amy. "The gap between yourself and your desires is like a buffer that deadens feeling. Feeling your way out of boredom is the only solution.

"If you are honest in your search for your own feelings, you will hit upon love, even if it is only the tiniest spark of attraction and desire. Some hint of desire must be present no matter how numbed a person may be. Instead of deciding that these faint impulses are too insignificant to act upon, take the opposite tack. Put your newfound feelings at the feet of your beloved—express kindness in the smallest of ways, praise even the humblest quality, smile outwardly when an inner smile flickers. In this way you encourage a fragile new emotion to believe that it is legitimate, that it has a right to exist."

For the first time in our talk, Amy looked encouraged. "Fred doesn't really know that I still love him," she said, sounding very vulnerable.

"And asking him to read your mind isn't going to work," I said. "The web of tenderness that once connected you has been torn, but it can be rewoven, I promise."

From this starting point—"I love you"—the channels of passion gradually open up. The relationship that seems to frustrate and kill desire turns into the healer of desire.

"I have a special name for the kind of healing I'm asking you to try," I said. "It's called 'wooing the goddess.' What you ultimately want isn't Fred or a better sex life. You want the return of spirit within you, which is the return of God. The passionate side of God is Shakti, the goddess. Passion was the wedding gift she brought when she married Shiva. It is also the gift women bring to men today, for the female principle is desirable by nature. It excites consciousness with arousal and yearning. It melts opposites into union and makes chaos into a dance. It was your birthright to be that passion."

"You make it sound like I could be," Amy said, actually laughing for the first time.

"If you don't feel at one with the goddess," I said, "woo her back. Win her before you try to win anyone else. Go into the fear and hurt; practice letting go of your old beliefs; learn to forgive yourself; find moments when you can be kind to your inner being; claim what is good about yourself and not just what is bad; follow every enthusiasm wherever it leads you, since the source of enthusiasm is always passion.

"Spirit is waiting for you to rejoin her. She stands outside the boundaries you have imposed on yourself. There is no passion too great for her to contain; you will never be lost reaching for the infinite. She is the tenderest of infinities, whose only desire is to protect you and carry you in her arms from fear to love."

# 7

# ECSTASY

What we have discussed so far is how to ground a relationship in love through surrender, nonattachment, and the renewal of passion. When two people have found such a basis of lasting love, they are ready for the next stage on the path, which we can call ascension. Ascension is based on love's ability to expand beyond the world of limitations to the world of boundlessness. Before ascension "I" refers to a single individual isolated in time and space. After ascension "I" refers to a self that observes time and space without feeling trapped by them—you have slipped through a sliver of time to find the timeless. Before ascension "you" meant someone who could be loved but never merged with. After ascension "you" means a part of oneself who is as close as breath. Before ascension "we" meant a couple who met in mutual need. After ascension "we" has no meaning, since union is complete.

Ascending is a process, like falling in love or being in relationship. You are not carried away into the "other world." This world becomes transformed into a heaven of fulfillment, ever at peace, ever in love. The process of ascension doesn't call upon anything new

from inside you other than letting go and letting go until there is
nothing more to let go of; ascension is the final stage in relinquishing
attachment to separation. Someone who is ascended has achieved
Christ's injunction to be in this world but not of it.

*As you ascend, your love will turn to ecstasy.*

To feel ecstasy is the privilege of all who have walked the path
to this point, where ascension begins. If you have not yet come this
far, ecstasy is not within your normal range of feeling. You may
know joy, delight, exuberance, satisfaction, and happiness, but these
are shadows of the ecstatic state. It exists as an ideal that is more or
less unreachable through any emotion the ego can grasp.

The fact that ecstasy takes us beyond ego is implied in the roots
of the word itself—in Greek *ekstasis* means "to stand or place outside." One can read this in two ways. Either ecstasy requires you to
move outside yourself or it is standing all around, waiting to be
noticed. There is more than a subtle difference here. Do you have to
go someplace to find ecstasy, taking an extraordinary journey into
unknown realms? This is what mystics and poets seem to do, fetching
back their ecstatic experiences like precious cargo from an exotic
land. Or is ecstasy so close that we miss it because no one has shown
us how to touch it?

*Ecstasy is the final stage of intimacy with yourself.*

Before ascension intimacy is achieved by reaching out to someone else. Reaching out implies a gap, and what we have learned so
far is that this gap, which appears to be between "me" and "you," is
actually inside each of us. Therefore what lovers really heal when
they love intimately is the relationship with themselves. Throughout

time you have been seeking to love yourself, heal yourself, forgive yourself, and find God in yourself. All outer relationships, which come and go in time, serve this eternal relationship. Eventually your seeking is done. A moment comes when you experience a merging, as Emily Dickinson so exquisitely describes it:

> The Drop that wrestles in the Sea—
> Forgets her own locality—
> As I—towards Thee.

This is the crystalline instant in which pure love fuses into pure religious devotion, for ecstasy overpowers all separation; ego gives way to pure flow of being.

To be in ecstasy permanently is known in Sanskrit as *Moksha,* which is usually translated as "liberation." It could just as correctly be called ascension, for arrival at the end of love's journey identifies you with the pure observer, witness, and seer that has been with you every step of the way, just above and beyond the world of ego and its needs. Moksha ends karmic bondage; it abolishes individual memory, desire, and identity in the cosmic ocean. Yet in some mysterious way liberation is not an extinction or annihilation but a new birth, a birth into fullness. When moksha comes, the individual has three distinct realizations:

> I am That,
> Thou art That,
> All this is That.

These simple statements, first enunciated thousands of years ago in the Upanishads of India, are the most intimate revelations that spirit can impart to humans. The word *Upanishad* derives from a Sanskrit phrase meaning "to sit close by," referring to how near one must draw to God in order to understand these teachings.

*"I am That"* is the first revelation. It abolishes all separation between the soul and God. This is the moment when the drop dissolves into the ocean, when a person looks at all the good and bad things in his existence, the struggle between light and dark, the contrast of virtue and sin, and sees them all as equal. Everything that mattered to the mind is reduced to a play of the Being within itself. "I am That" means "I am Being and nothing else."

*"Thou art That"* is the second revelation. It denotes the sacred nature of the beloved, for "Thou" is both God and lover. In this revelation a bridge is built between two souls; there is no possibility of separation because the perception of "I" melts into the perception of "Thou." Two truly breathe as one; the celestial vision of the Creator becomes personal. One can gaze like a loving parent on every person.

*"All this is That"* is the third revelation. It is an expansion of the first two revelations to encompass every particle in the universe. This expansion delivers total unity as the individual ego finds that it is actually cosmic ego. "I" is no longer an isolated speck, a viewpoint bounded by time and space. Instead of feeling that I inhabit a body, I sense myself as infinite consciousness expanding with infinite speed through infinite dimensions.

These three strokes of moksha require extreme purity and refinement of awareness to be sustained. The greatest masters and saints throughout history have been capable of this liberation; it is the quest each of us undertakes when we step onto the path to love. Without ecstasy the experience of liberation might seem impossibly distant, given its incredible magnitude. At the end of the *Bhagavad-Gita,* Lord Krishna, who has been posing as a chariot driver to the warrior Arjuna, agrees to show himself as he really is. He opens his mouth, in which appear all worlds and creatures, infinite universes expanding so rapidly that the mortal Arjuna reels on the verge of extinction.

Yet all that moksha represents is a shift in awareness, a final perception of who we are. Therefore the insights of ecstasy have much more to do with the final expansion of consciousness than with any feeling or emotion, however remarkable.

> *Ecstasy carries you completely outside your ego boundaries.*
>
> *In ecstasy you know yourself as cosmic ego, unbounded in time and space.*
>
> *The end of love's journey returns to the source of all aware-ness, power, and being.*
>
> *Moksha is not an ending but a beginning—we begin to live in fullness only after liberation.*
>
> *A liberated soul is a citizen of the universe.*

There is really no adequate equivalent for moksha in Western culture; *redemption* may be the closest synonym. Moksha unites self and soul in the mystic marriage that in Christian terms is union with the Redeemer. Angels are said to be in this state, which gives rise to their ecstatic praise of God. The difficulty with redemption, how-ever, is that it is generally a future state, realized after death; therefore it is much more mystical than moksha, which can be achieved here and now.

## DREW'S STORY

Having said that liberation is like a new birth, I'd like to relate the story of someone who went through that birth, my mystical friend

Drew. *Mystical* is a term that has been attached to Drew since the day we met. It was at a meditation course years ago, and Drew attracted considerable attention. He wore a white Indian dhoti, sandals, and more chains of beads than I had ever seen on a yogi in the Himalayas. When everyone gathered in chairs before the outdoor stage for presentations, he sat in lotus position under a grove of trees on a nearby hill. I'd never met anyone who had a foot more firmly planted in the "other world," and his talk was an outpouring of mind-boggling experiences of astral planes and angelic visitations. When I last heard of Drew, he was in Nepal, having taken vows in a monastic order deep in the mountains. In some ways I felt jealous of the life he had chosen.

Then one day he called me and asked if we could meet. He appeared at my door sans beads, sandals, and dhoti, dressed in a sports shirt and chinos. We talked, and I quickly found out that, unlike ten years ago, Drew now never visits psychics or readers of any kind and in fact feels total indifference toward paranormal phenomena. "I haven't sold out on all that," Drew said. "Something deeper took its place." He proceeded to tell me about a breakthrough experience he had had, one so powerful that it had changed his life.

"You don't know me very well, but I've always been ambitious, fiercely so, some people would say. I fought to get into the best prep school, the best college, the best fraternity. I don't remember how I hooked up with the idea of mysticism and enlightenment—maybe an old girlfriend or a trip on LSD—but once bitten I wasn't going to give up until I turned into something magical—sorcerer, warrior, seer, psychic, and prophet if I got that far.

"It was all rampant ego, as I look back on it now, but at the time my experiences were pretty fantastic—I had the lights, the bliss, the angelic voices, and while it was all happening it never occurred to me that what I was experiencing was actually one and only one thing: my expectations. Mysticism was high drama, with me at the center lapping it all up. We're talking about ten years of extraordinary visions. Then one day I was in Vermont, walking up a perfectly green hill, when it all collapsed.

"It was like being sucked down a drain. My head started spinning, and I had to sit down. I couldn't tell if I was plummeting down a hole or if the earth was sinking out from under me. It was a terrifying sensation. I had a sudden horror of turning around, for I expected to see the sky opening into a funnel that would suck out the world. I closed my eyes and lay down, praying that whatever this was would just end.

"It took about an hour. I might have passed out during that time—I didn't have a watch on—because even when I felt like I was coming back to reality, my head buzzed. I got up, still extremely wobbly, and walked down the hill to my cabin; the dizziness didn't fully go away for several days, and I continued to feel disoriented. What do you make of that?"

I had been listening to Drew without comment. "Well," I said, "if a patient came to me with that kind of experience, I guess I'd suspend judgment until we took a brain scan and ran a psychiatric profile."

"Bingo—either I was dying of a brain tumor or I had suffered a psychotic break. That's exactly what I told myself. I ran to the village library and madly scanned some old medical books. The thing was, I didn't have double vision or any return of severe dizziness. I didn't have disordered or racing thoughts. The clinical explanations for this episode didn't seem to apply. Gradually my symptoms vanished, but not without a trace.

"I was different. It was as if someone had pulled the plug and drained out my—what? Battery fluid. I didn't have any charge left; no ambition, curiosity, purpose, drive. I was pointless to myself, and my mystical experiences had disappeared completely. If I shut my eyes to meditate, there wasn't any light; I didn't expand outside my body or see angels. For a few days afterward I felt extreme anxiety, as though demons were going to get me, but that didn't happen either. So if it wasn't tumors, madness, or divine punishment, what was it? I waited for an answer."

"Did you get one?" I asked.

"Yes, but not the way I expected. The answer was a process, which I began to call 'ego surgery.' That dramatic moment on the mountain was like having my chest opened up by an invisible surgeon, and once opened I couldn't close myself up again. It hadn't occurred to me, in my headlong pursuit of the never-ending high, for that's what spiritual life had meant to me, that spirit is carved out of the very things a person doesn't want to face. Like most people, I wanted not to be sad, anxious, powerless, unlovable, and hostile. I wanted 'It,' the big spiritual payoff. But what I now got was every speck of sadness, anger, anxiety, and so on that I thought I had gone beyond."

"It must have been a difficult time," I said.

"To put it mildly. Whoever this surgeon was, he dug deep, probing for every hidden secret, every dark deposit of guilt and shame. There were mornings when I felt that nothing could be worse than simply living with myself. But I got used to what was happening, once I realized that the surgeon was me, working on myself. At some deep level I had given myself permission to go through the dark night of the soul.

"Ironically, I'd always thought that getting to God meant climbing a mountain, getting so close to Him that He would say, 'Ah, you've made it, I see.' With a smile of approval He would then grab my hand and pull me into heaven. There's only one problem with that scenario. What happens to the parts that get left behind? I certainly didn't expect God to say, 'Bring along your shame and guilt.' To me, being spiritual meant jettisoning the 'bad' me and boosting the 'good' me to heaven."

"But that would imply," I said, "that God judges against the 'bad' you and only loves the 'good' you. Such a God couldn't be a God of love. He would be a God of ego, since that's exactly what our egos do all the time—judge against the bad and accept only the good."

"Exactly," said Drew. "I suppose that's why ego surgery was so difficult to face. Once these awful things—the ghosts in the basement, I call them—were exposed I actually had to take them back. You can't imagine how disgusting that seemed at first. I mean, all our dirty secrets look hideous in our own eyes, no matter how common they might appear to others."

"I don't think it's the horribleness of the unconscious that is the main block," I suggested. "It's more our fears about forgiveness. What you're talking about is forgiving yourself so that you can take back your dark energies and turn them into love. What if that fails? What if you're stuck being as ugly, dirty, sinful, and undeserving as your worst judgments say you are? That prospect is so terrifying that even tiny sins and blemishes get expanded into monstrosities."

Drew nodded and sat still for a moment. "There were times when I didn't think I was going to make it. A voice inside kept crying, 'You're going to die. You can't take any more.' But I knew I wasn't going to die. My spiritual life had taught me at least that much. I went back to my old job as a stockbroker, and so far as I knew nobody had any idea of what I was going through."

He noticed my amusement at the kind of job he had chosen. "You like literature, I recall. Didn't Hawthorne write somewhere that a man may go around to all the world looking like any other man while entertaining the most extraordinary ideas in his head?"

"In his journals, I think. But that could apply to psychotics as well as visionaries," I said.

"True, but my point is that something that appears normal can be very wild inside. Which had not dawned on me when I was running around trying to become a visionary. I walk down Milk Street with my briefcase, and I ask: Is a tree a tree, a skyscraper a skyscraper? What makes these things 'normal' is that they look like separate, solid objects, but they're not. They're bundles of energy carved out of the infinite energy soup of the universe, and so are you and I. Therefore at some level you and I are not simply connected with that tree and that skyscraper. We *are* that tree and skyscraper. And that is what a mystic knows, nothing else."

"You have closed the gap," I said, feeling both moved and impressed.

"Something like that. Have you ever sat by a river, all alone, and tried to feel it? Of course you can't. You may say that you're feeling the river—its flow, its still depths, its constant change that runs unopposed from here to there—but all you actually feel is yourself. If you can get close enough to it (and such feelings are very tough to get close to), the sweetness of sitting by a river actually comes from a tiny point in your heart. That point of sweetness is perfectly still; it doesn't reach out for you, but it doesn't ever abandon you either. What's in that sweet point?"

"Everything," I said.

"Yes, everything."

We both sat without speaking, relishing this moment of communion. Then Drew said, "The ego surgery ended. At a certain point the process spit me out. I can't say I did anything, really, but in some way I had been through the crucible, and now, past the flames, what was I? I was real. It's astonishing to realize what a difference it makes to find out that you are not false, since to the rational mind *of course*

I am real. It's a given. But to really be real, that's the joy. That's the revelation. That's the ecstasy."

Impossible as it is to convey ecstasy through the poor power of words, we can sense what it is, because all of us live from that sweet point in our hearts. Whatever seems to be happening on the outside, every person wants to hold on to that spot forever. It is touched in love, sometimes in sex, often in moments of supreme creativity. When we succeed in getting there permanently, the transformation goes beyond self to change the world.

*Ecstasy makes this world into God's world.*

The certainty of one's divine status is probably the most important gift ecstasy brings, as evoked by Whitman in his poem "Song of Myself":

> I know that the hand of God is the elderhand of my own,
> And I know that the spirit of God is the eldest brother of my own,
> And that all the men ever born are also my brothers
> . . . and the women my sisters and lovers.

These words came from a direct, undeniable fusion of self and love. The melting sensation that ushers in ecstasy isn't meant to be temporary; when you remain open to spirit you become spirit, and then universal love is your natural state. It's true of all lovers that at moments of intense joy some sort of boundary melts, and the happiness of loving another person is exalted beyond itself. One crosses over into a place where the traces of personality diminish until they become so faint that the ego merges into love's flow like that drop returning to the ocean.

Despite the fact that only a small percentage of people may have fallen in love on any given day, lovers have not taken extraordinary journeys, not compared with those mystical travelers often called ecstatics. The intense joy of romance is a reachable experience, a step on the same path that mystics travel much farther along. Now it is time for us to see what the final destination actually is.

## VARIETIES OF ECSTASY

Rather than use a vague term like *mystical,* we will explore the different experiences that have been labeled ecstatic throughout history. Ecstasy can first be considered as a *physical* experience. This is the level our culture has fixated upon, to the extent that a drug has been given the name Ecstasy with the promise, presumably, that it will deliver the experience. In the very crudest sense pushing sensual pleasure to its limits is supposed to bring one to the point of ecstasy. Books on erotic technique pass themselves off as handbooks to the ecstatic.

But in all these cases the real nature of ecstasy has been missed, because no lasting transformation has taken place. A drug may alter the brain's biochemical status, mimicking the spontaneous sensations that appear in ecstatic states, but the experience is devoid of meaning. Altered brain waves do not equate with the poetic insight of this exalted passage from the Song of Solomon:

> My heart was split, and a flower
> appeared; and grace sprang up;
> and it bore fruit for my God.

These lines are supremely sensual, the images are undeniably sexual. Yet the poet is not mistaking his ecstasy for mere pleasure, however deep and intoxicating that may be. He declares,

> And my drunkenness was insight,
> intimacy with your spirit.

Without this insight ecstasy might justifiably be equated with sensory intensity such as drugs can deliver. Here my intent certainly isn't to strip the pleasure away. Lovers who can freely surrender in sexual intimacy are able to go far beyond the experience of partners who feel inhibited with each other. Pleasure is by no means a given in a society that has not yet really confronted the guilt and shame that cloud sexual desire. Yet the boundaries that melt in the experience of ecstasy are of a different kind. As the most famous lines from the Song of Solomon declare,

> And you have made all things new;
> you have showed me all things shining.
> You have granted me perfect ease;
> I have become like Paradise.

For all things to become new and shining requires much more than sensuality. If anything, intense sexual contact leads to release and exhaustion; the "little death" of orgasm is a form of oblivion, not a raising of consciousness. We can't afford to be absolute here. Sexual energy is neutral; we mold it according to our own intentions. For some lovers it is possible to use orgasm as a means to reach elevated states of consciousness, yet even in these cases the visions, sensations, and emotions being evoked are not necessarily ecstasy. They are whatever the lovers have made them into.

To make things shining and new has everything to do with perception. This brings us to the second broad definition of ecstasy, which is *mythic* or *archetypal*. In ordinary perception we see ourselves in unmythic terms, overshadowed as we are by so much mundane activity. Ulysses didn't have to commute through tangled traffic every morning; Athena's mind wasn't filled with worries over meeting the mortgage this month. But as Carl Jung long ago pointed out, beneath the turmoil of daily activity our unconscious motivations dwell in the mythic world.

Inside each of us are primal gods and goddesses. We know this without knowing it, insofar as we obey our mythic drives without bringing them into conscious awareness. Striving to succeed in a corporate takeover bid partakes of the heroic quest as much as the Argonauts seeking the Golden Fleece; climbing Everest is driven by the same ambition to reach the abode of the gods as Icarus flying toward the sun. In mythic terms ecstasy is a sacred journey into the unconscious as underworld, heroically portrayed in countless ways, from Persephone's abduction by Pluto to Orpheus seeking his bride among the shades of Hades.

If the physical definition of ecstasy falls short because it lacks meaning, the mythic definition flirts with being too intellectual. Through the arduous process of bringing the unconsciousness to light, a person may be able to reach his mythic roots, but whether this will bring ecstasy is questionable. In the language of archetypes ecstasy has been traced back to the Greek god Dionysus, whose devotees engaged in ritual orgies, using wine and sexuality to attain altered states. At the sacred site of Delphi, a secret cult of women called maenads (derived from the Greek word for "madness") worked themselves into ecstatic frenzies in their rites, which included skinning animals alive with their bare hands and devouring them.

We still look askance at Dionysiac revels, supposing that their participants reached wild excesses of drunkenness and promiscuity. To mythic thinkers, though, nothing could be further from the truth. The worship of Dionysus, they tell us, was not about excess and violence but about the attainment of divine ecstasy. The darkness of this journey is what made the frenzies necessary; they were not an end in themselves. In any event, orgies are now really grand metaphors for smashing the shell of waking consciousness to arouse the sleeping divinity within.

Perhaps this is true. Many ancient traditions use extreme states to push through to sacred visions. Native shamans who pierce their bodies or seclude themselves in the harsh wilderness are attempting to contact primal forces within. Their rites and the orgies of Dionysus are not that far removed from lovemaking by lovers who hope to push sex into the intensity of ecstasy. The transports of priests and devotees through devotional rituals can be very meaningful to them. The unconscious is a rich landscape; archetypes tell us much about our primal selves. Yet the messages of myth often seem prefabricated, I think, lacking the immediacy of true ecstasy. It is rare to meet a mythic thinker who has recaptured the divine states of the ancient ones he or she has thought about.

## True Ecstasy

This brings us to the third definition of ecstasy, as a *spiritual* release. Spiritual ecstasy is not a feeling or an idea but a shift of perception in which direct contact with spirit is made. Being in ecstasy does not have to express itself through intensity of any kind. The biblical injunction "Be still and know that I am God" is an invitation to ecstasy.

I prefer the spiritual definition because it is inclusive of the physical and the mythical. The most famous example of spiritual ecstasy is probably that of Saint Teresa, who dreamed that an angel came and pierced her heart with a golden arrow. She describes this experience in intensely physical terms, as a burning pain that was almost unendurable until it wondrously transformed itself into equally intense pleasure. The mythic ingredients of the angel and the arrow are unmistakable once we think back to the god Eros with his quiver and bow. In her ecstasy Teresa felt nothing less than the intimate embrace of God, and the erotic and mythic overtones of her experience make it no less divine. Being supremely spiritual, her ecstasy is able to include every level of interpretation.

What usually makes ecstasy so intense and extreme is not the experience itself but getting to it. The common images of God or an angel coming down from heaven to pierce, shatter, and penetrate the ecstatic one do not have to be taken literally; they serve to remind us that many layers shield us from contact with spirit. To receive the gift of ecstasy is an exquisite experience, as told in a remarkable passage from a Greek Orthodox manuscript written a thousand years ago:

> For if we genuinely love Him,
> we wake up inside Christ's body
>
> where all our body, all over,
> every most hidden part of it,
> is realized in joy as Him,
> and He makes us, utterly, real.

These sensual lines, which aroused shock and controversy at the time, were written by an obscure monk known to us as Symeon the New Theologian. His description of spirit as a penetrating, transforming love that turns our very cells to divine essence still may sound too intimate for comfort:

287

We awaken in Christ's body
as Christ awakens our bodies. . . .

I move my hand, and wonderfully
my hand becomes Christ, becomes all of Him. . . .

I move my foot, and at once
He appears like a flash of lightning.

Symeon was well aware that his loving intimacy with Godhood would be considered blasphemous—he spent his last years exiled in a remote Turkish village, condemned by church authorities—but now we can recognize in his writing the complete sincerity of a true lover. For Symeon "everything that seemed to us dark, harsh, shameful, maimed, ugly, irreparably damaged, is in Him transformed and recognized as whole, as lovely, and radiant in His light."

This of course sounds like the voice of a saint, and a very ecstatic one. But I believe the same vision is open to us all—we are all lovers trying to reach perfection. We do this, as Symeon teaches, when "we awaken as the Beloved in every last part of our body." In Symeon's time these words violated the dogmatic belief that the body was wicked and corrupt. In our age the opposite prejudice applies: a lover is someone whose appeal is basically physical, sexual. In both cases the fusion of spirit and body has been missed.

Yet at moments the piercing joy of love does appear, despite dogma. The touch of your beloved or simply the sight of her can seem suddenly amazing, appearing like lightning, just as Symeon says. But the same feeling can penetrate the heart from nowhere, because love is inherent in life itself. Emily Dickinson, whose lovers were all in her imagination, is to me a true lover nonetheless. She writes:

# Ecstasy

Not "Revelation"—tis—that waits
But our unfurnished eyes—

This is a message of compressed wisdom, which says that we are waiting not on the day of redemption but on our own perception.

The exquisiteness of true ecstasy cannot dawn unless we can contain it; our minds are so absorbed in relentless activity that quietness rarely lasts more than an instant. The body by its nature is also active and restless. Since activity and stillness are opposites, the body generally registers some degree of agitation or even discomfort as it moves into alignment with spirit. The reputation that ecstasy has for being physically intense contributes to the frenzy and mutilation that devotees have resorted to in order to duplicate the opening to ecstasy—they are mistaking the symptom for the cause.

The divine has nothing to do with pain. Because it stands outside—*ekstasis*—the envelope of time and space, spirit cannot be sensuous. Our five senses cannot take us to where ecstasy dwells. But as true ecstasy begins to manifest, our senses definitely react. The reaction is entirely individual and unpredictable, since one person's intense erotic opening is another's frightening collapse of defenses. What feels like the expansion of the soul into infinite space to me may seem like a terrifying fall into the void to you.

When we say that ecstasy is like the drop melting back into the ocean, it must be made clear that we are the drop and the ocean at the same time, just on different levels.

*Ecstasy is the release of individuality back into wholeness. Whatever brings you closer to wholeness brings you closer to ecstasy.*

Here I think we've reached the secret of ecstasy. Most of us do not see ourselves as supreme sexual technicians, nor can we relate easily to the extraordinary mysticism of a saint. Ecstasy will never be ordinary, yet it can be brought within our reach once we realize its real nature. Although often experienced in the most extreme situations, ecstasy is a quality of spirit as natural as any other. We do not have to sojourn into the darkness of the mythic past to retrieve it. The patient work of inner growth is all we need.

To promote stillness inwardly is to promote ecstasy. The inner being doesn't have to be tricked or manipulated to achieve this stillness. Our minds are like runners that only have to slow down in order to walk, then slow down from a walk to standing still. This process of shifting from activity to stillness is a simple yet very deep description of meditation. We could modify the biblical injunction to "Be still and know ecstasy." There is no single road to this quietness of meditation, yet to be genuine any meditation must take the mind beyond its superficial nature, which is restless and chaotic, to its deeper nature as the peace that passes all understanding.

## REACHING ECSTASY

The emergence into stillness can take place under any conceivable circumstance. Arjuna achieved his moksha on a raging battlefield after the bloody onslaught of family against family. Medieval saints found theirs in complete retreat from the world. At this very moment someone is finding it in a bustling city or staring out to sea. The release is never incidental or accidental. Tastes of ecstasy come and go, yet attaining complete stillness of the mind means walking the spiritual path to its conclusion, with discipline and faith.

*Expansion of consciousness is the road to ecstasy.*

Expansion of consciousness is a broad term that covers almost everything I have discussed up to now, for the path to love is all about such expansion. Love pulls you out of ego boundaries, and when you are dedicated to acting from love, you are able to live in spirit. Many of the most important themes have already been covered:

> Seeing your beloved as a mirror of your higher Self.
> Surrendering to love as a guiding force.
> Letting go of attachment to the false self and its needs.
> Devoting every day to achieving true union and healing
> the wounds of separation.

Countless people live with their beloved without following any of these principles; their love doesn't provide a strong enough basis to escape their old conditioning. Until they discover the spiritual path, few are able to heed the voice of spirit, which speaks intuitively. If only you perceived it, you are already in a state of ecstasy that is permanent and unshakable. But only at moments when your boundaries fade away do you have flashes of reality. Then direct intuitive knowing becomes possible, and you can see yourself for who you are, sublime and ecstatic. Thousands of years ago the Upanishads expressed our twofold nature in a beautiful metaphor:

> Two birds, one of them mortal, the other immortal,
> live in the same tree. The first one pecks at the fruit,
> sweet or bitter; the second looks on without eating.
> Thus the personal self pecks at the fruit of this world,
> bewildered by suffering, always hungry for more,
> but when he meets the true Self, the resplendent God,
> the source of creation, all his cravings are stilled.

The two birds in the tree, self and Self, are inseparable; both sit in the same tree (the body) faced with the same fruit (the material world). Yet for all their closeness the bird who craves the fruit does not know its mate. It takes an awakening to reveal the Self, and although in one sense it is awesome, being "the resplendent God," in another sense it is just one's intimate beloved, who has faithfully kept watch through all time, waiting only to be seen. Once it is seen everything in life changes. As the Upanishads declare, the life of the self, once united with the Self, rises to a blessed level:

> Good and evil both vanish;
> delighting in Self, playing like a child with Self,
> he does whatever is called for, whatever the result.

When self-realization dawns, there is no longer any question of struggle or effort. The spirit guides you to do whatever is called for, according to your own makeup. In reality universal love requires only one thing, that the sweet point in the heart expand until bliss and peace become the nature of our life. This first happens within individuals, then it happens to relationships based on spirit, finally it extends to whole families and societies.

*A single point in the heart can expand to liberate the world.*

Ecstasy is therefore not an individual feeling at all but a glimpse of the wholeness waiting to be seen everywhere. The Upanishads state this very explicitly:

> Self is everywhere, shining forth from all beings,
> vaster than the vast, subtler than the most subtle,
> unreachable, nearer than breath, than heartbeat.

Our senses tell us that we are breathing and that our hearts beat, but there is a breath within the breath that is spirit (in Christian terms it has been called *afflatus,* the breath of God).

Near as spirit may be, centuries of cultural prejudice have made it necessary to rediscover our intuitive, direct knowledge of it. Many disciplines and techniques can be employed here, particularly meditation. In this book I have concentrated on the expansion of consciousness that is available through love, motivated by the tragic absence of love we see all around us. Yet the road to the Self is not closed on any side—the transcendent is "nearer than breath, than heartbeat"—and fortunately a multitude of teachings exist to put our feet on the path.

In the end the path does not actually ascend anywhere in time or space. The self is still the self, the ego is still the ego, the senses are still the senses. How can you go anywhere to capture what is already so close to you? The mystery is that this "pathless path," as the masters refer to it, causes immense transformation. There is a world of difference between those who live in love and those who only touch upon it fitfully. Perhaps the greatest difference is this quality called ecstasy, which is the actual feeling of breathing God's breath and beating with His heart.

I do not want to betray the intimacy of ecstasy; it is the most private of love affairs. Being becomes your beloved, and the merging of yourself with another person follows with complete ease and naturalness. If one had to lay down some kind of pattern for how ecstasy is attained, it would be extremely general, as follows:

The time comes when seeking is over and realization begins. First the mind becomes aware of its own activity while standing apart from it. Ordinarily we are immersed in our own inner dialogue; the stream of thoughts, wishes, fears, and fantasies running through our heads keeps us fixated. We buy into a mental drama that has no conclusion. The mind gains its restless energy from our participation.

Being fixated on your own mental drama is all it takes to cause the drama to work itself up.

At certain moments, however, the fixation is not so alluring. Some part of ourselves detaches from the mind's activity—the first stage of ecstasy is just this faint awareness of being a witness to the drama rather than an engaged participant. The observer has begun to put a slight distance between itself and the observed.

The second step is the stilling of the mind. This is not achieved by force or indeed by any action at all. Doing anything is the opposite of being still. Because we have spent our whole lives in activity, non-doing is extremely unfamiliar. Most of the time it occurs by accident —out of the blue, one notices that the stream of consciousness has ceased, like turning off a water tap. Sexual activity is so often associated with ecstasy because it is one of the few times that most people can be fully distracted from their minds. Whether a person tries to make it happen or not, what creates stillness in the mind is simply that the ob- server is able to continue to stand apart for longer than a moment.

Gaining some distance between the observer and the observed is so rare that the second stage of ecstasy occurs quite infrequently. For most of us the excursions away from mental activity last only a few seconds. But if we manage to achieve the second stage, stillness takes on a surprising aspect. Our attention reveals to us that silence has its own dynamism. The still mind, though devoid of thoughts, quivers and vibrates all the same. There is a kind of trembling anticipation that can go one of two ways. Either a new thought will be born to bring back the internal dialogue or the faint trembling of silence will lead to even deeper silence.

Poised here at the edge of ecstasy, you cannot make your mind choose one way over the other. Even people who have experienced silent mind many times, such as in prolonged practice of meditation, do not go past the front room of silence at will. But if the mind chooses to plunge into deeper silence, the third stage has been reached. This deeper silence doesn't quiver; it cannot be disturbed by even the faintest activity. One experiences it like the softest black velvet or the deepest dark cave. Anyone who has come this far is now truly "standing outside." Of course it would be just as accurate to say that you are standing inside, because inside and outside have lost their difference. You are merely there where ecstasy is.

The fourth and final stage requires nothing new on your part—once your attention has been captured by deep silence, the inner transformation is complete. Whatever is to happen next dawns of its own accord. One is brought face to face with pure Being, pure awareness, pure joy. In ancient Sanskrit terms, *sat chit ananda,* eternal bliss consciousness, reveals itself. A Christian saint might call the same experience "the face of God." The poet of the Song of Solomon put it in lover's terms:

> My eyes are radiant with your spirit;
>> my nostrils fill with your fragrance.
> My ears delight in your music,
>> and my face is covered with your dew.

But these are images only. The fact that ecstasy exists is the promise that kindles our faith on the path to love; tastes of it are the water that refreshes our quest. We take faith from those living masters who have reached the goal. They stand apart from us, yet they are clothed in the same flesh and bones; they move, act, breathe, and live as the rest of us do. Only secretly, in their realized souls, do they know with utter certainty that, like the two birds in the tree, they are Self while we are self.

I often turn to a few pages of dialogue between an Indian disciple and his master that bring this contrast to life for me. The disciple is resisting the idea that there is anything beyond the world of the senses. He is the questioner; the answerer is the South Indian master Sri Nisargadatta Maharaj:

Q: Is your world full of things and people as is mine?

A: No, it is full of myself.

Q: But do you see and hear as we do?

A: Yes, I appear to see and hear and talk and act, but to me it just happens, as to you digestion or perspiration happens. . . .

Q: If you are the world, how can you be conscious of it?

A: Consciousness and the world appear and disappear together, hence they are two aspects of the same state. . . . As long as the mind is there, your body and the world are there. Your world is mind-made, subjective, enclosed within the mind, fragmentary, temporary, personal, hanging on the thread of memory.

Q: So is yours.

A: Oh, no. I live in a world of realities, while yours is of imaginings. Your world is personal, private, unshareable, intimately your own. Nobody can enter it, see as you see, hear as you hear, feel your emotions and think your thoughts. In your world you are truly alone, enclosed in your ever-changing dream, which you take for life. My world is an open world, common to all, accessible to all. In my world there is community, insight, love, and real quality; the individual is the totality. . . . All are one, and the One is all.

As many times as I have read this passage over the years, it never fails to move me at a level deeper than emotion or memory or even insight. I feel brought face to face with the real, and I stand in awe of a person who can say of the material world that it is the merest speck fleeting through his mind. But it is also heartening to realize that such great masters began as ordinary people. The only difference between them and any one of us is that the masters set foot on the path, beginning the journey of soul-making that leaves time behind. Eventually the path ends, and the foundation of our world, which stands upon memory and mind, crumbles, leaving a new world of unimaginable realness. Understandably, Maharaj's disciple was intensely curious about what this new world is like, but his master could only answer him from a place beyond words:

Q: How do you know that you are in the supreme state?

A: Because I am in it. It is the only natural state.

Q: Can you describe it?

A: Only by negation, as uncaused, independent, un-related, undivided, uncomposed, unshakeable, unquestionable, unreachable by effort. . . . And yet my state is supremely actual, therefore possible, realizable, attainable.

There may be those who would find this a discouraging description, riddled with paradox. How can the unreachable be reached or the indescribable be real? I can only turn to those arrows of light that hurtle at us from that world, the moments of ecstasy that quiet all doubt and still all questionings. It takes a long time before such experiences born in the deepest silence can be translated into time and space. A life filled with chaos is extremely difficult to fill with ecstasy. While you are caught in the ecstatic moment, however, all of reality seems like a miracle. The very root of the word *miracle* reminds us that it derives from the Latin *mirare,* "to behold with rapt attention." No better definition of ecstasy has ever been given.

To those who have gained entry to ecstasy there is no reason to ask for more. No transformation is as all-embracing, and after returning to the everyday world, the great gift seems to be not the intensity of remembered joy but the revelation of truth. One moment of genuine ecstasy removes a lifetime of doubts—you realize once and for all that spirit is real. You know from firsthand experience that you are the divine essence. In that sense ecstasy is the most immediate and yet the most far off of experiences. It is immediate because it is undeniable; it is distant because it will take a lifetime to secure ecstasy as a permanent reality. Fortunately this journey itself creates ecstasy, being the path to love.

# LOVING PRACTICE

## Cultivating Inspiration

One of the most beautiful proofs of ecstasy is delivered in a moment of inspiration. I have already discussed signals from spirit which hint at a reality beyond that perceived by the five senses. But inspiration is much more than a hint—when you feel inspired you find yourself thrust into a world where ordinary objects and events are full of light, as if illuminated from within. This inner light is truth, and when we suddenly see the truth, we gain insight, clarity, and objectivity.

> Insight enables you to know your own heart.
> Clarity enables you to accept without illusions.
> Objectivity enables you to view any person or situation
>    with compassion.

At triumphant moments when you say to yourself, "That was really inspired," all three qualities come together, and the *feeling* of that union is ecstasy. Sadly, most people do not attain even a few of these qualities until late in life, when the maturation of experience allows the obstacles to inspiration, particularly fantasy, projection, and judgment, to fall away. Even then moments of inspiration may be rare. But the root word of *inspire* means "to breathe in," which implies that inspiration should be a simple thing—as natural as breathing. When we say that someone has been inspired to write a love poem, we mean that it flowed naturally from his or her feeling; nothing stood in the way. There was no struggle between mind and heart.

*Inspiration is that state in which mind and heart are connected.*

The following exercises show you how to summon inspiration and make it your own long before you reach the end of the path.

### PART ONE: AN INFINITE MOMENT

Every spiritual master has declared that the present moment is the home of spirit; nothing to be attained in the form of wisdom, love, and vision has to be postponed Yet we all postpone the day when we will be loving, wise, and inspired by our own vision. This implies that the present moment is a very difficult place to reach, despite the obvious fact that we are already there.

*Every second is a door to eternity. The door is opened by perception.*

What makes each second infinite is its potential; what makes it finite is your view of that potential. Think of an inspired moment in your life, when you made the perfect move, said the perfect thing, had the perfect idea. What made you so different in that moment?

You were open to something new.
You weren't reliving the past or anticipating the future.

You felt optimistic and open; you were not defended.

You let it happen, whatever it was.

You felt connected.

Now ask yourself if you feel that way *now*. If you did you would be in a very simple, though extraordinary state: you would be in the moment.

The same preconditions take everyone into the moment, whether Leonardo, William Blake, or just an ordinary person like me or you. A genius like Blake may see "infinity in a grain of sand," whereas an ordinary person might only feel uplifted and carefree. The differences, however, are much less important than the similarities. If you doubt that you could actually see infinity in a grain of sand, try the following meditation (which can be done imaginarily without sand, in case none is handy).

Hold a grain of sand—ordinary aquarium or beach sand will do —in the palm of your hand and let your eye rest upon it. Notice its color and facets, any hint of glitter, the sharpness of its edges. Roll it between your fingers; hold it up to your tongue to taste if there is saltiness or earthiness in it. This is the grain of sand presented to you by your five senses, and most people would say that there is not much to see in this humble object.

Now think of your grain of sand as a point surrounded by space. How much space can you imagine? There is the room you are sitting in, which expands out into your house, the house into your neighborhood, neighborhood into town—allow your mind to see this expansion suddenly explode. Now there is the space of the whole planet, the solar system, galaxy, and blackness beyond. Let this space also expand, and allow yourself to see that there is no edge to outer space, no boundary in time. Space cannot have a boundary because the cosmos is expanding at a tremendous rate, hundreds of thousands of miles per minute, which is barely slower than the speed of light in human terms. You cannot take a stop-motion picture of the cosmos to find out where it is right now, because at the leading edge of expansion, the universe curves back onto itself. It must do this; otherwise there would be something *outside* space, which cannot be.

> *This means that your grain of sand is the center of the universe.*

Now repeat the meditation using time instead of space. Look at your grain of sand and check the exact time. Imagine the earlier part of the day stretching before and the rest of the day stretching after. Now expand the time frame to include a day before and after, a week, a month, a year. See time as an expanding circle and allow it to expand as fast as it wants. Is there a limit to this acceleration? In your mind you can instantly envision the moment of the Big Bang; I don't mean the literal event, which is beyond mental comprehension, only the time it takes you to bring the event to mind. Likewise, if you want to imagine a star as it exists 10 billion years from now, your mind can go forward to that point instantly.

> *Your grain of sand is the center of time, expanding infinitely in all directions.*

If time and space both are centered on one grain of sand, then you have seen infinity—or as close as your present perception can carry you. The next step is to perform this meditation without the *idea* of time and space. Let your mind go blank and allow the sensation of time and space, a single expanding circle, race away from a point. Hold in your mind both extremes—the point and the circle

—without letting go of either. Don't strain or try to visualize too hard; this should be as natural as possible. Let the circle race away from the point until it disappears and you can no longer hold both things in your awareness.

Sense the state of your mind:

> Is it open, watching, and alert?
> Is it reliving the past or anticipating the future?
> Is it undefended?
> Did you let your meditation happen, without turning it
>     into something?
> Do you feel connected?

You may notice any or all of these things—or none. This isn't a test but a way to go beyond boundaries. The value of seeing infinity in a grain of sand is personal: you may feel like laughing or you may feel profoundly quiet, you may have a beautiful image come to mind or a silky emptiness, you may be ecstatic or inspired. Give it some time —this meditation opens the mind, easing your old ego boundaries without your having to address them psychologically.

The grain of sand is important. You are using this point of focus to slip out of the net of time and space. Beyond the net lies openness, which is pure potential. In that potential everything is possible. It is the door of the present moment, which leads to eternity.

## PART TWO: THREADS IN THE FABRIC OF LOVE

On the path to love, inspiration grows. The moments of insight that mark the early stages of the path are not as profound as those that come with mature vision. This reflects a change of consciousness, but at the same time there is a change of reality. Being infinite, spiritual reality is infinitely flexible. It can accommodate any perspective. All perspectives are valid, yet those that approach nearer to God contain more of His qualities: truth, compassion, acceptance, and love.

> *Your consciousness is your contribution to reality. What you perceive as real becomes real.*

When two people come together in love, they weave a fabric of consciousness. If the fabric is strong, then both lovers have made it so; each loving thought and action is a thread added to the fabric. In Sanskrit the word for "thread" is *Sutra,* which also has a metaphysical meaning. A sutra is an aphorism or formula that expresses some fundamental truth about consciousness. When Rumi says, "Love is the sea where intellect drowns," he is uttering a sutra. It expresses a truth from his level of awareness, and at the same time it weaves truth by adding a thread no one else has added before. In a moment of clarity and insight, Rumi felt within himself that his intellect no longer struggled against love but was absorbed into it, as if being drowned in the sea. His sutra reflects that experience and at the same time evokes it in us as we read it.

You and your beloved have privileged moments in which you understand what your love is. No one else has ever had exactly the same revelations, because you are unique people. Your inspirations are yours alone, even though similar insights have been occurring for thousands of years. To make your revelations your own is important. You need to know what you believe, how far you have come on the path together, how much growth you have shared. Sutras can tell you all these things.

The exercise here is to write down your inspirations as they come to you. Love grows the more you talk about it, think about it, and express it. Even though moments of insight last only an instant, they are touchstones of something eternal, the relationship between self and Self. At this moment your Self wants you to know about love but also about truth, compassion, trust, acceptance, and devotion. These are the threads from which the fabric of consciousness is woven.

### Writing sutras.

Get yourself a notebook in which you will put your sutras, as well as record those of others that inspire you. Do not wait to enter only your inspired thoughts. At any moment spirit is ready to teach you about itself; you only have to set aside some time when you feel receptive—taking five or ten minutes in the early morning works for most people.

Sit down with your pen and paper, and let your mind relax. Do not force yourself into a state of inspiration, but have the intention to express *what you know*. I don't mean the information in your brain but what you know from your heart—a spark of truth, a message from your Self. If words don't come so easily at first, you may want to start with a standard opening, such as "Love is . . ." or "My Self wants me to know that. . . ." After a little practice, however, you won't be able to stop writing—once communication starts, it tends to pour out.

The purpose of your sutras isn't to sound poetic or wise but simply to express where you are. Most of us cannot equal the brilliance of Rumi, but our state of awareness is just as true for us as his was for him. The beauty of recording your spiritual vision is that you will have the immense pleasure of watching it grow. Each thread is valuable; none can be taken out of the fabric of love without loss. Therefore keep in mind the preciousness of your own awareness, and let your inspirations be a way to claim your spiritual life as your own.

# THE PATH *to* LOVE

The following are some sutras I have written over the past year in my own notebooks. I wrote them in spare moments, on airplanes, waiting for lost luggage, or sitting outside by the sea on sunny days when I wanted to be with my Self and hear its voice. There are nearly a hundred sutras here, a good harvest from a very busy year, and I was surprised, once I read them all, how completely they express the material in this book. Thus they are like crystals from which whole pages sprouted and grew. I do not offer them for you to read in one sitting, but all are given here to mark the progress of one soul as it unfolded over a short span of time. If I could wish one thing for myself, it would be that I weave this fabric of consciousness forever—what is more thrilling than the prospect of truths you do not yet know?

## LESSONS FOR LOVERS

Three things are absolute and cannot be destroyed:
awareness, Being, and love.

You will be in love when you know that you are love.

Love is the impulse of evolution that expands life.

Any desire to grow is following the flow of love.

If you block your desires, you block your natural avenue of growth.

Growth is the willingness to let reality be new every moment.

# Ecstasy

Love is the beginning of the journey, its end, and the journey itself.

The path of love is everywhere and nowhere. There is no place you can go that is devoid of love and no place you can leave that is not already love.

Love is based not on how you act or feel but on your level of awareness.

In duality love comes and goes; in unity there is only love.

Personal love is a concentrated form of universal love; universal love is an expanded form of personal love.

Loving another person is not separate from loving God. One is a single wave, the other is the ocean.

The mind judges what is good or bad. Love brings only good.

All prayers are answered. The ones answered the fastest are prayers for understanding.

Desires are fulfilled according to your level of awareness. When awareness is pure, every desire is fulfilled completely.

A prayer is a request made from a small part of God to a large part of God.

Dreams come true when they are held quietly in the heart.

Don't tell your dreams to the world—whisper them to love.

# THE PATH *to* LOVE

From a pure heart, anything can be accomplished. If you ask what
the universe is doing, it is eavesdropping on your every desire.

Everything is the same spirit watching itself through
the eyes of different observers.

Love is everywhere, but in some places it is blocked by fear.

What does not contain love must contain an illusion.

Pierce through all your illusions and you will discover that
you are only love.

Other people are mirrors of your own love. In reality there are no
others, only the Self in other forms.

Separation is merely an idea. At its core, reality is unity.

When you blame and criticize others, you are avoiding
some truth about yourself.

Everything in the outer world contains a message about
the inner world.

The sights and sounds of nature are reminders of a loving creation.

Real change is accompanied by a new insight.

Insight is an impulse of love dissolving some old imprint.

Insights bring truth, which is love in action.

# Ecstasy

Love is like water. If it doesn't flow, it stagnates.

If you create any open space within yourself, love will fill it.

Contemplate love every day. Loving reflections make
the heart grow.

Love takes many forms—it is up to you to choose
which you wish to express.

The highest expression of love is creativity.

Innocence is the ability to give and receive love without
holding on.

To love innocently is to allow others to express who they are.

No one is wrong. In the eyes of love, all people are doing the best
they can from their own levels of consciousness.

Other people seem wrong when their perspective doesn't
match yours.

All disagreements are results of misunderstanding
someone else's level of consciousness.

All obstacles are created by ourselves, through a belief in non-love.

You will have no enemies once you decide to surrender.

Surrender means not giving in to another but giving in to love.

# THE PATH to LOVE

All desires are spiritual when seen to their deepest level.

Love is not the opposite of hate. Being whole, love has
no opposites.

Negativity is born in the gap where love has been excluded.

Gaps occur in places where we are afraid to see ourselves.

Life appears random on the surface, but at a deeper level
it is completely organized.

Love's organizing power is infinite.

The cosmos is structured to bring about growth, and growth is
always in the direction of greater love and happiness.

The solution is never at the level of the problem—the solution is
always love, which is beyond problems.

Bad things don't happen to us; we bring them to us
so we can learn a lesson.

Love grows on the basis of giving.

God's ability to give is infinite. We limit it by our own
unloving perception.

Love never forces. Love is intelligent and brings only what
you need.

# Ecstasy

There is no divine punishment. What seems like God's punishment
is a reflection of our own resistance.

Forgiveness is born of increased awareness. The more you can see,
the easier it is to forgive.

Forgiveness in the heart comes about when the
walls of separation in the mind fall.

Love is attention without judgment. In its natural state,
attention only appreciates.

The person you call an enemy is an exaggerated aspect of
your own shadow self.

The shadow self seems to be the opposite of love.
Actually it is the way to love.

Spirit is passionate; without passion no one can be truly spiritual.

The awakening of true love lies in finding peace within passion
and passion within peace.

Sexual energy is neutral. It can be loving or unloving,
depending on how you use it.

Sex can be used to expand love or to shut it out.
The highest eros is to take God as a lover.

When sex is fully loving, you experience the divine through
your partner.

# THE PATH *to* LOVE

Sexual love, energized by absolute love, is ecstasy.

Ecstasy is the most primordial energy state.

Why is sex so powerful? Because we are constantly in search of the state of original ecstasy.

The whole of reality is contained in the present moment.

True love is here and now. Whatever you can remember or anticipate is only a shadow of love.

To see love in the moment you must clean the windows of perception.

If you have your full attention in the moment, you will see only love.

When love is replaced by an object, the result is addiction.

If you are addicted to someone else, you are treating that person as an object.

Time is the ego's enemy, not love's.

Love changes with the passage of time, but it never diminishes. It is always present in its fullness.

Love is the eternal Being at the core of individuality.

# Ecstasy

Love can create a world that is healed and holy.
The two are the same thing.

To feel beauty is to know the truth. To know the truth is to
be in love.

Love dances in the freshness of the unknown.

Love doesn't need reason. It speaks from the irrational wisdom of
the heart.

A heart that has learned to trust can be at rest in the world.

# IN OUR LIVES

## A House of Light

"I think every couple starts out wanting to belong to each other—it's only natural, isn't it? I mean, we're born belonging, until we wander off."

Elise's voice spoke through the half darkness. The three of us—Elise, her husband, Kent, and I—were sitting outside in New Mexico. The long light of sunset had made the hills stand out in blue shadows, ridge after ridge that filled with gold and then emptied again.

"The whole question of love is finding where you belong," Elise went on. "It's never been easy for me, and even when I met Kent I wondered where we would end up."

"Not a hopeful way to begin," I said. Elise laughed.

"We started out with a hideous honeymoon. That's what we both called it. Rushed plans, total disagreement over where to go, and when I finally gave in to Kent's dream honeymoon, which was in Paris, we spent the first two nights stranded in a snowbound airport outside Chicago. After such a start, wouldn't you worry?"

"It must have gotten better," I said.

"Yes and no." It was Kent's voice this time coming through the darkness. "We had anticipated working together at our own small business, but when we got out here, the economy slumped. I wound

314

up spending most of my time uselessly at home while Elise worked a counter job in town. It was the worst time to be apart, and the longer I found myself out of work, the more depressed I got. It was all pretty unlivable."

"They say you can't live on love alone," Elise remarked. "God knows we tried, but you bring so much emotional baggage with you when you marry. Particularly us, since we'd both been single until our forties. We were extremely hard to please, like the grocery store cat."

They both laughed. You would never suspect, five years later, that anything like a hideous honeymoon or the troubles that followed had ever happened to this couple. I have rarely met two people who seem so genuinely to belong to each other. The first thing that strikes an observer is that Elise and Kent have learned to turn love into play. Their eyes sparkle when they look at each other; they laugh easily and find endless sources of interest in their life. Their home in the New Mexico desert is crammed with folk art, each piece purchased from an artist Elise and Kent personally trekked to find in an exotic country.

It was disarming to enter this home, so full of light that at times I could hardly tell it had walls. Every object had a story or a name. Ambrose was a carved wooden armadillo six feet long from the highlands of Guatemala; Matilda, a shaggy coyote sewn from brown velvet, sat at the dinner table looking absurdly gentle. Everything in their environment represents an extension of how these two people love.

"If I tell anyone about you," I said, "you will come off as dangerously close to the perfect couple."

"We're not afraid to claim what's good about us," Elise said. "Being fifty entitles you to that."

"We just know how to survive," Kent put in.

"Meaning what?" I asked.

"Like Elise, I went through a lot of years when belonging to someone else was hard. Part of this was personal—I really had no idea what an intimate relationship meant, and getting close to anyone frightened me. But I was also caught in the cross fire of a culture that expects a man to be hard when he's outside his home and soft and romantic when he comes back at night. Love and power are hard to mix."

We took this as a line of departure and talked about it for the next few hours. "I agree," I said. "But I think it's about more than just being hard or soft. There's a spiritual issue here. Human beings are the only creatures born with a higher nature and a lower nature. At different times one may suit the situation better than the other."

"Define *higher* and *lower.* Those terms make me nervous," Elise said.

"In the West *higher* and *lower* are equated with sacred and profane, that part which is close to God, and its opposite, which lives among the animals. Sex, being profane, is lower; love, being sacred, is higher. But in fact sex and love are processes—they are ways of feeling and doing.

"In India it's taught that the same life force, or *Prana,* runs through everything. In Christian terms Prana is the 'breath of God,' which transforms dead, inert matter to life. But even though Prana is the same energy wherever it flows, it gets colored. As sex the life force is not the same as when it is love."

"But why call these *higher* and *lower?*" Kent asked. "Is it lower to make love to someone than to give alms to the poor? Love is love."

"Ideally, yes. If you could just be in the flow of love, distinctions wouldn't matter. But as everyone finds out, if a man loves his job and devotes every waking hour to it, his wife doesn't consider that enough to compensate for his absence; the lack of love on one side is still painful. So the question is, how do you restore love on all levels?

"First, you'd have to know which levels we are talking about. For thousands of years in India it has been taught that humans live on seven levels. These are visualized as seven wheels or *chakras* arranged up the body, starting from the lowest chakra at the base of the spine and ending with the highest at the top of the head."

None of this came as news to Elise or Kent, who had read a good deal of metaphysics. "Will this really get us to love?" Kent asked. "Not many people in the West are going to plunge into esoteric knowledge, are they?"

"That's not where we have to head with this," I said. "If you skip the details, all that is being described here is a simple division between the higher and lower energies. The bottom three chakras are located below the heart. They have to do with survival, sexual drive, and a sense of power. If we only lived in these three chakras, human beings would be fierce, self-protective, instinctual creatures.

"Above the heart are the three higher chakras, devoted to will, intuition, and freedom. If we only lived from these centers, human beings would see themselves as divine. We would never go to war, struggle for survival, or create enemies. So why is our nature divided in such a radical way?

"The answer lies in the heart, the chakra that stands midway between higher and lower. The heart is the mediator, the chooser, the center of feeling. It looks upon the higher and lower energies, and its response is always the same: it loves both. The function of the heart isn't to label anything good or bad; it doesn't judge or reject. Out of love it blends high and low until something new is created: a complete human being, totally at ease with every aspect of himself."

"So why do we struggle so hard?" Elise asked. "Your scheme has a beautiful symmetry to it, which in my experience means it is probably totally unworkable."

"Who can really say?" I replied. "The problem is that so few people ever get to test whether they can marry higher and lower. Our society, to be brutally frank, is stuck in the bottom two chakras. Sex and survival dominate our awareness. We laud the power brokers but rarely the men of peace; we judge the powerless as weak and inferior, and we hand out few rewards for spiritual achievement."

"That sounds pretty accurate to me," Elise said wryly.

"This imbalance is reflected in the way aggression and violence still come forward to solve problems, which means that the lower chakras have been threatened," I said. "When anything is threatened, it gets activated; that's just how life works. So how does a person activate the higher energies? What would it take to end a war with compassion? The answer is actually simple: human beings will act out of their higher nature when they become complete. What we call human today is really half a person.

"The only way to become complete is to call upon your heart to start blending higher and lower. It won't do any good to shove violence and aggression out of sight, or to pretend that we can be loving without facing those dark areas in the psyche where fear and insecurity constantly prowl."

It was night now, and the sky was full of stars in brighter splendor than I ever see from the city. I stopped talking, waiting to see how this perspective would be received.

"I think I know where you're going," Kent said. "The heart brings together two opposite energies, as you call them, until they have no choice but to face each other. Then what happens?"

"Only one thing," I said. "You have a relationship. Instead of living in two separate worlds, the high and low must look at each other. Isn't this what happens in marriage? You bring all of yourself under another person's gaze, and you see the same in return. You become mirrors to each other, and when you look in those mirrors, what you see is sex, survival, will, emotion, purpose, and love. It's all there, but it isn't whole. The fragments don't completely fit, therefore you get conflict and pain."

"Isn't that inevitable?" Kent asked. "Love is about surviving the wounds another person can inflict and feeling bad about the ones you inflict in return."

"Of course that is inevitable," I said. "But the question is why we want to expose our vulnerable, fragile, conflicted selves to someone else. Why look in the mirror? The view, after all, can be quite brutal."

"You look because you want to love," Elise said.

"Exactly. The mirror of relationship gives back love, not all the time or in all love's purity. But the reflection is there, every day. Here's what I think happens in every relationship where love is alive. The energies that make us act out of anger, fear, insecurity, and doubt are extremely familiar. They are like an old, dark house we return to whenever things get too hard to handle. It feels risky to leave this house and see what's outside, yet we have to leave if we expect to be loved.

"So we take the risk. We walk out into the light and offer ourselves to a beloved. This feels wonderful; it's like nothing we ever imagined in our old, dark house. But when things get tough, we run back inside; we choose the familiarity of fear and lovelessness over the vulnerability of love, until finally we feel safe enough to go back and try love again.

"This is essentially the rhythm of every intimate relationship—risk and retreat. Over and over we repeat this rhythm, accepting love and pushing it away until finally something miraculous happens. The old, dark house isn't necessary anymore. We look around, and we have a new house, a house of light. Where did it come from? How did we build it? It was built from the love of the heart. It has silently been weaving our higher and lower natures, blending fear, anger, survival, and protection into the energies of devotion, trust, compassion, and acceptance."

"And that's when you belong to someone else," Elise said. "You feel safe enough to live in love together, without retreating into the old, dark places."

"Yes," I said. "If two people come from love, no matter how much they have to overcome, eventually the house of light will be finished. This is the project silently undertaken in all intimate relationships. The tragedy is that our culture doesn't teach us to see love and marriage in this way, so not enough people ever finish their house."

We sat quietly, our talk nearly done. I had never really spoken like this before. I felt a warmth of gratitude that these two people had created a safe place for such words to emerge. Words are fragile when tied to tender emotions, and to find oneself in a place that nurtures the fragility of love is rare.

"If you really love someone else," I said, "you are not afraid to let that person look in the mirror you hold up. There is no other way to grow. And you are not afraid to claim your share of love in return, because you have looked in the mirror too. The ultimate mystery of love is that by looking deeply into yourself, you find out who you are, but then that self is given away, offered in love.

"I do not want to give half of myself to my beloved. Therefore I must find my completeness. To find who I really am, I must get in touch with spirit in everything—in moments of silent meditation, in the beauty of nature, in the practice of nonjudgment, in appreciation of this precious instant in time. I must see my life as a work in progress. Nothing about me is ever final.

"Knowing that my path is the search for love, I have to devote some time every day to this search. I must place my beloved above myself in order to deserve a vision of her sacredness. I must tread lightly on the path, having patience with setbacks and harming no one who seems to block me. I must experience my shadow and learn from it in order to go beyond it.

"I must see all things in myself, rejecting nothing out of fear or disdain. I must remind myself always to look a little bit beneath the surface of things, for a flower is not just a flower—it is rain and rainbow, clouds, earth, and the immensity of space. Then I must look at myself the same way.

"All of this is how we build a house of light. A faint voice calls us from outside our old, dark house. It says, 'Can't you see the vastness in your heart? Don't you perceive that you are enough, needing no one and nothing? What could be more desirable than being here and now, savoring the infinite in the moment?' Just to heed this voice for a second is to experience love. To listen to it forever is to experience all of life in the light of love. Then what we lay at the feet of our beloved is a treasure, the treasure of who we really are."

"I'd like to think that we have built a house of light," Elise said. She had gotten up to go to the kitchen. Kent caught her hand in passing, and I'm sure they exchanged smiles in the gently gathering night. They were not afraid to own the best part of themselves, which is always true of people who have learned to live from the heart.

# IN CONCLUSION: "YOU ARE LOVED"

"Can I help you?"

Hearing the woman's voice, I looked up from the mess of glass, water, and soggy paper littering the floor. Hundreds of people had been rushing by to catch their planes, and I didn't even want help. "I can take care of it," I said.

"No bother, it'll only take a jiff," the woman said. She opened her purse and produced, miraculously, a towel. She knelt down and started dabbing around on the floor. I had dropped a carry-on bag in the airport and smashed a bottle of mineral water. The exploding glass had ripped the flimsy nylon, spilling the bag's soaked contents onto the floor. All I could find to clean up the mess was toilet paper from a nearby men's room.

"That's getting it," the woman said. "It wasn't as bad as all that."

"You're English, aren't you?" I asked. She nodded and smiled. "My name's Laurel." As she efficiently finished up, I had time to take a long look at Laurel. She was plain-looking with pockmarked cheeks and frowsy brown hair, wearing no makeup and a gray stretched-out cardigan. We both stood up, and I saw her wince slightly. I took the towel and threw it in a trash receptacle by the men's room. Laurel nodded slightly as I thanked her, and when I offered to walk her to her gate, she hesitated, again very slightly.

"That would be nice," she said. We gathered our things and headed up the concourse. I couldn't help but notice that she had a decided limp. "A very unbeautiful woman," I thought, "and very kind." I wondered what made Laurel the way she was. When she got to her gate, it turned out that the flight to London had been delayed for half an hour. We began to talk.

"I'm just going home to see my mother," Laurel said. "She's getting on, and she's not so cheerful as before. Osteo and the rain. It's what she must live with, I suppose."

"Do you go home often?" I asked.

"Me? No, not in twenty years, if I count right." I must have looked surprised. "Well, they didn't really want me at home. I left the first day it was legal to drop out of school. My family's working class, and after my leg was hurt—I was riding on my boyfriend's motorbike—they just found it too hard having me around. Natural, I guess."

Something in me was feeling very pained. "They threw you out, you mean, because you were crippled?" I asked.

"That's a bit dramatic. I just use a cane when I have to." Laurel's recitation of these events had been given in a calm voice, free from bitterness.

"So what made them decide to take you back now, after all this time?" I asked.

"They didn't, exactly. I just want them to know, well, what everyone needs to know." I looked at Laurel, whose face became eager; she had decided to tell me something special. "A very remarkable thing happened to me recently. I went to a women's conference being held up in the mountains. I live in New Hampshire, doing child care and the odd thing or two to make ends meet. A woman whose child I take care of couldn't go to this conference, which was at quite a lovely resort, so she offered me her place. I decided to go, just on the spur of the moment. So you see, I didn't even belong there with the others."

"That's important to what happened next?" I asked.

"You're a good guesser. I liked being in the mountains and having such a nice room, but the rest of it, the discussion groups and such, frankly went over my head. Only the last night did I work up the courage to go to one, and what do you think? They asked us to close our eyes and imagine a very sad day in our past. It was some kind of emotional therapy, I think you'd call it. So I closed my eyes and imagined the first day I was sent to school. I must have been five, and I cried so hard they couldn't get me to let go of my mother's skirt. She was fussing and telling me not to be such a baby. I think she was quite embarrassed by my carrying on like that.

"Then they told us to open our eyes and pick out any stranger in the room. We were to walk up to her and exchange experiences. I plucked up my nerve and picked out a woman about my age in the corner. I told her my experience, and her eyes grew wide and strange."

I had a sudden premonition about how this story would turn out. My skin tingled, but I held my tongue.

"She almost stammered telling me her own experience," Laurel said. "And what do you suppose? *It was exactly the same as mine.* Then I asked her, 'You're from England, too, aren't you?' and she nodded. 'I'm Vicky,' she said, all excited. 'Don't you remember me, Laurel?'

"I stood back, quite amazed. Then I did remember: there had been another little girl just as frightened as I was that day, crying her eyes out. 'Do you mean to say we had the same experience? You were going to find a stranger to tell it to?' I asked. Vicky nodded, and we didn't know whether to laugh or cry. Imagine!"

"It's an amazing coincidence," I said.

"No, it's an amazing *reminder.*" Laurel replied. "You see, I had been getting discouraged, being alone and without my family. You can see how it is. And here this astonishing thing happens, and I realized that I couldn't possibly be alone. You do see?"

I had to suppress the emotion in my voice. "Yes," I said. "As amazing as your experience was, the really remarkable part to me is that you know what it's about."

"Oh yes," Laurel said. "It's about God. It has to be."

There is nothing more moving than a reminder that spirit is with us. This woman had been gathered into a web of delicate caring that encloses all of us, though we do not notice it. Rumi was being quite literal when he said,

> There is someone who looks after us
> From behind the curtain.
> In truth, we are not here.
> This is our shadow.

The tragic illusion of everyday life is that we mistake shadow for reality. It is impossible to be outside the web woven of love, and at moments when events throw us too far into oblivion, a message comes to say, "You are loved."

"So you've decided your mother would like to know that she's not alone," I said. Laurel nodded. "But you don't owe her anything," I said.

"I owe her everything," Laurel said. "It's just that people forget if the debt lasts a long time."

"Does it matter that she's had so little care for you?"

"How do I know that?" Laurel asked, surprised. "Perhaps she can't show it."

It still amazes me how often spirit sends us clues about the real nature of life. This I took to be a clue about compassion, the closest value to love itself. To be compassionate is not to take pity; it is to extend care to others simply because you see their need. Most of us give because doing so increases our self-image or because we expect something in return, although it's difficult to be entirely honest about that. Laurel gave *because she had to*—this is love in action, having no doubt about itself. There is no question of anyone else having to deserve your compassion. If you have it to give, you will give it where it is needed.

The path to love doesn't end with ascension, as if that were a fixed and final stage. Ascension continues as long as you live. Through ascension the ideals of trust, forgiveness, devotion, and compassion ripen into a golden harvest whose seed was planted years before in our first lessons on love. And whatever aspect is revealed at a given moment, they ripen because they have to.

"A lot of people would say that you have a right to be bitter," I told Laurel.

"They're probably people who are bitter themselves," she said casually. We parted company at her gate, and for some reason I noticed that she was carrying one of those dilapidated paperback thrillers the British dote on. "That book says a lot about you," I remarked, smiling.

"It does?" she asked.

"Yes. It says you like to look for clues."

I went off to my flight, but this unusual woman has stirred me to write about compassion as the last thing I have to say in this book.

I don't think compassion is very well understood. In the West we have been misled by the word itself—the Latin roots of *compassion* mean "to suffer with." Yet compassion does not have to entail suffering alongside someone else. To be in touch with God's love is the root of compassion. Trying to exercise compassion without this connection will only lead to failure. If I see you in extreme distress, putting my attention on your suffering is the same as participating in it, and the amount of love I can actually direct to you will therefore be diminished.

Compassion, to be full, has to be founded on unconditional love, which is not attached to suffering of any kind. I think of all the conditions that could have held Laurel back—her physical limitation, the injustice of how she had been treated, her obvious lack of money. But she was on that flight nevertheless, to deliver the message "You are loved."

The remarkable thing was how equally Laurel saw herself to others she might have resented. Compassion, besides being connected to God's love, sees everyone as connected to it in the same way. Even if you are presently in pain, you are not without love. Since God is compassionate, no one's experience of pain is a punishment. There is love somewhere inside. Suffering is hard to perceive as love when it is occurring, and many times it isn't perceived as a lesson for growth either.

This is where compassion has most value; it allows me to step in and remind you that you are loved, not in theory but in the flesh. All of us feel our pain keenly while the pain is present; there is little room for reflection on the spiritual value, if any, of what we are going through. But the fact that the mind is dominated by pain doesn't negate love's purpose. A time will come, a state of awareness will grow, that transcends the suffering. Spirit will dominate the mind instead. By bringing compassion to you, I can reassure you that you are not abandoned; you are just at a difficult crossroads on the journey of love.

At every stage of love the goal should be kept in mind. Uniting romance, relationship, and ascension is a code of compassion, which goes as follows:

> Be kind to yourself and others.
> Come from love every moment you can.
> Speak of love with others. Remind each other of your
> spiritual purpose.
> Never give up hope.
> Know that you are loved.

If you practice these few things, you will be open to receive every lesson on the path in the spirit in which it is given—as an expression of divine love. The horrors of the world are undeniable, and few people even dream that they will go away. But they will, because love is the supreme reality, compared to which all else is temporary, fleeting, and unreal.

The love you seek is seeking you at this moment. Your longing, your deep fantasies about being loved are mere shadows of the melting sweetness that makes spirit want to love you. Be honest about your seeking, and be alert to the moments when love is showing itself to you. You are the only means that love has for conquering its opposition; therefore you are infinitely precious in the eyes of spirit. The messages of love may not be clear to anyone else around you, even those most intimate to you. That doesn't matter; they are meant for you and you alone. Be assured of that.

And above all, be like Laurel. Keep looking for clues.

# INDEX

# Index

# Index

Surrender, 156–88, 189
  and being in love, 4
  and commitment, 157, 159
  and dharma, 158–63, 166–68
  and ego, 156–57, 163–64, 168, 169
  and faith, 156
  and falling in love, 164, 165
  loving practice, 169–78
  and marriage, 162–63
  and need, 164–65
  in our lives, 179–88
  to passion, 134
  to the path, 157–58
  in a relationship, 158–63
  and sex, 136–37
  to the spirit, 160, 161–63
  struggle against, 165–66
  and "the Way," 163–68
Sutra, 304–13
Sutras, writing, 305–13
Symeon the New Theologian, 287–88

Tagore, Rabindranath, 131–32
Tao, 161
Teresa, Saint, 286–87
Thou art That, 275
Tolerance, 203
Transcendence, 92–93, 94
Transformation, 293, 295
Trust:
  and courtship, 109–11
  and marriage, 160

Truth:
  vs. falsity, 111–16
  inner, 38
  and knowledge, 11–12
  in phenomenon, 97
  spirit as, 97
  Veda as, 11

Unity:
  and attachment, 191
  and healing, 43
  and love, 35
Unreality, and false love, 113–14
Upanishads, 274–75, 291, 292

Veda, 10–11
Vedic scriptures, 10–15, 36, 195, 225–26, 242
Vishnu, 243

"The Way":
  and surrender, 163–68
  Tao as, 161
Whitman, Walt, 103, 105, 217, 226, 282
Will, 242
Willingness, 59–60
Wordsworth, William, 89–90, 91
Worship, and bhakti, 35, 36, 87–88

You are loved, 322–28

338

# ABOUT THE AUTHOR

Deepak Chopra, M.D., has established a distinguished career as writer, lecturer, and physician. He is the author of sixteen books and thirty tape series, including the breakthrough bestsellers *Ageless Body, Timeless Mind* and *The Seven Spiritual Laws of Success*. He has made five television specials for PBS, including *Body, Mind, and Soul,* and most recently *Alchemy* and *The Crystal Cave*. Beginning in 1996 he has headed the Chopra Center for Well Being in La Jolla, California. He lives in La Jolla with his wife, Rita.

Deepak Chopra and Infinite Possibilities International offer a wide range of seminars, products, and educational programs. For additional information, please contact: Infinite Possibilities International, 60 Union Avenue, Sudbury, MA 01776, U.S.A. 1-800-858-1808 (toll-free)/(508) 440-8400. For medical inquiries and health-related programs, please contact: The Chopra Center for Well Being, 7630 Fay Avenue, La Jolla, CA 92037, U.S.A. 1-888-424-6772 (toll-free)/(619) 551-7788.


*The Path to Love* is also available as a Random House AudioBook, read by the author, and in a large-print edition.